Hey, Doc

The Wonder of Animals
from the Life-stories of a Texas Vet

David Carlton, D.V.M.
&
S.E. Christine

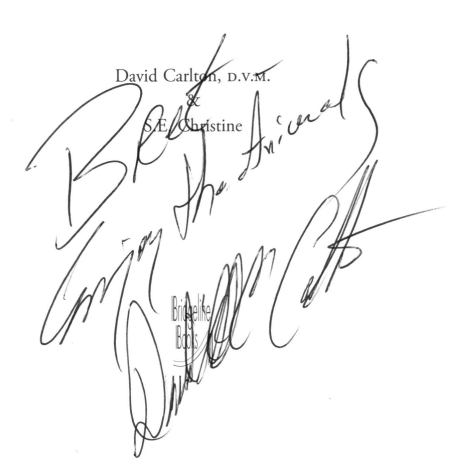

Bridgelike
Books

HEY, DOC: The Wonder of Animals from the Life-stories of a Texas Vet.
Copyright © 2006 by David Carlton and S. E. Christine. All rights reserved.
Printed in the United States of America. No part of this book may be
used or reproduced in any manner whatsoever without written permission
from the publisher, except in brief quotations within articles or reviews.
For orders and information, contact publisher: BridgelinePress@aol.com
or phone 800-585-1488.

Disclaimer: To ensure privacy, all names and dates have been changed
and reported events altered. Neither the authors nor Bridgeline Press
shall have any liability or responsibility to any person, group, or entity
with regard to alleged references or similarities to actual persons or
events, created directly or indirectly, by the stories depicted herein.

FIRST EDITION

Designed and produced by Graffolio, La Crosse, Wisconsin.
Printed by Hignell Book Printing, Ltd., Winnipeg, Manitoba, Canada.

*Cover artwork from an original pencil drawing entitled 'True
Companions'. Copyright © by Sheri Greves-Neilson. Information and
other works can be seen on the artists's website (grevesneilson.com).*

Library of Congress Cataloging-in-Publication Data

Carlton, David, 1949-
    Hey, Doc: the wonder of animals from the life-stories of a
Texas vet / David Carlton – 1st ed.
      p.cm
   ISBN 1-888843-05-5 (pbk.)
     1. Carlton, David, 1949- 2. Veterinarians – Texas – Dallas –
Biography. 3. Veterinary Medicine – Texas – Dallas – Anecdotes.
I. Title.

SF613.C37 A3 2006
636.089'092—dc21
[B]

2005058268

To my wife, Karen, and son, Kyle

And to our clients, four-legged friends,

and veterinarians…everywhere

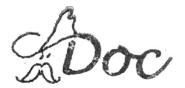

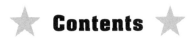

Contents

1

Kitchen Vet

Wherever a vet finds himself...at a party, picnic, or shopping and, yes, even mowing the lawn ...people will come by with questions about their pets. Even our local Maria's Pizza spot isn't sacred anymore. But since the welfare of their animals is as important to me as it is for them, I've never really minded. Generally, though, when clinic duties are over and I'm finally home, I like to think that all my concerned clients and furry patients are fast asleep. It doesn't work out that way.

A few months back, exhausted from a heavy day, I was about to fall asleep standing up when my wife Karen sent me off to bed. Thankfully laying my head on the pillow, I silently prayed for a full seven hours of repose. About 11:30, banging noises at our front door awakened us out of this blissful state. Sliding into my slippers and fumbling with the tie on my robe, I made my way down our dimly lit, drafty hallway, mystified as to why our dogs weren't having a barking fit.

"I'm comin'...I'm a comin'...who's there?" There was no answer. "Who is it...what do you want?" Again, no answer. So paranoid fellow that I am, I grabbed a pistol from the desk drawer and tiptoed to the door, moving aside the curtain of a corner window ever so slightly to peer outside. Goosebumps crawled up my spine as I tried to focus my sleep-filled eyes. Three shadowy figures moved out from the darkness and onto the porch. Mustering up a threatening voice, I shouted, "I'm holding a gun...so you better tell me who you are."

A girl's squeaky voice said, "Oh, Uncle David, did we wake ya?"

Snapping on the porch light, I now saw them clearly. Shoving his overcoat collar up around his neck, Karen's younger brother Don stood there with his two wild yahoos, Travis and Ashley. I couldn't even remember the last time these relatives came a calling. Stifling a yawn while trying to be halfway polite, I was still reluctant to open the door. Trying to keep warm, three-year-old Travis, bouncing on one leg, then the other, was hardly dressed for the cold night in just a white shirt and shorts. Ashley, on the other hand, looked like the spinning top off a jewelry box in a bright pink ruffled dress. This weird scene gave me a deja vu feeling of a Halloween 'trick or treat'. Ashley was the one to say, "I hope you weren't sleeping...can we puleeze come in, it's freezing out here."

There was no love lost between Don and me. And he never came around unless he needed something or wanted to borrow money from his sister. But having been taught to honor family, I opened the door and let the smiling, but shivering, threesome inside. As Don pushed the kids forward, he said, "We could come back at another time." I thought to myself...if that's the case, why are you even here? Travis and Ashley darted past me and down the hall toward K.C.'s room...hollering, "Is K.C. awake?"

The light flickering on in my son's room was answer enough. I waited for Don to deliver whatever message was so important that it couldn't wait. He stood there fidgeting with his starched collar, and brushing a piece of lint from the lapel of his gray, tailored suit—his favorite on-the-job attire since he landed a half-time position as a Wells Fargo loan clerk.

I intentionally refused to ask about the box he was precariously balancing on his hip. So, instead, I asked why his wife Sherry didn't come. He explained, with some embarrassment, that after they came home from attending the community opera, 'Barber of Seville', Sherry demanded that he and the kids take their cat "...to Uncle David's and tell him to neuter it."

"Are you crazy?" came Karen's voice from the bedroom. "Tonight?...it's almost midnight!"

These two siblings couldn't be more different: Karen took charge of situations, while Don whined about everything, and could easily be bossed around. When they were kids, she climbed trees, rode horses, and played basketball. Don, on the other hand, preferred staying clean and pressed at all times. He dressed and acted like an English royal, but without a matching royal dowry. It was no surprise that he and Sherry got together. She nagged him to death, slept until noon, and shared his belief that credit cards were 'collectibles'. Still I needed to remember they were 'family'.

Yawning for the umpteenth time, I not so diplomatically suggested, "Don, why don't you bring your furry friend to our new Meadow Creek clinic tomorrow morning?"

After a sudden burst of movement within the box, out popped a kitten's head from between the two loose flaps. There's no telling how long the little year-old cat had been inside. But he was anxious and panting nervously. His claws were timidly extended, and, in search of security, he pushed and rubbed his whiskers against my hand. Mostly black, with white paws and a white chin, there were two smudged blotches of red lipstick on his brow. Judging from the intensity of the prints, I figured Sherry might be capable of feelings after all.

Karen came tromping down the hall, obviously ready to take someone's head off. "Please, Sis," begged Don, "Sherry will kill me if we don't do this tonight. I've got Sylvester here now...and besides I've got to work tomorrow." He never gave a thought to the fact that Karen and I also worked.

But I reluctantly agreed, "Okay, okay...I've done this procedure hundreds of times. Why argue about it. It won't take that long. Besides this was Sherry's idea anyway."

All I wanted to do was forget about our intrusive kin and focus on Sylvester. Throwing an old windbreaker on over my flimsy robe, I went out to Ol' Blue to make sure everything I needed was in my medical bag. When I returned with the surgical kit, the whole clan was in the kitchen. Since the cat had been cooped up for so long, Karen tenderly placed him on the floor so he could stretch and sniff at his surroundings.

When K.C. politely asked if he and his cousins could watch the surgery, I knew Karen would be quick to say, "No, y'all can't watch."

Judging by the size of the manly jowls on the shorthaired kitten, I figured Sylvester had kept Sherry awake too many times with his nightly prowls. He had sown his oats more than once, and his constant hollering was too much for my impatient sister-in-law.

Images of performing a sterile procedure in the spotless surgery room of our new medical facility were gone. Karen had been at my side enough to know what I needed. She flipped the lights on to their highest intensity. When I went to the sink to scrub my hands, she muttered, "I still can't believe Don's gall. And just exactly where are you going to do this?"

After spreading a clean, white dishtowel on the counter, I handed her the now relaxed cat by the nape of the neck, and asked her to hold him a moment. With a quick poke, I injected Sylvester in his hind leg with a short-acting general anesthetic, and told Don to put him in our utility room and turn off the light. We needed to wait for the anesthetic to take effect.

"Karen, I'm going to snip Sylvester and this fiasco in the bud, if not your brother first." Don flinched at the remark, and we couldn't help but snicker at his awkwardness when he tried to handle the still frisky kitten. He was never a 'cat person', and just the thought of getting hair on his immaculate duds unnerved him. Sylvester squirmed and hissed at Don, until K.C. grabbed the cat with his usual confidence, "Here, Uncle Don...give him to me...I'll take him to the utility room." And as soon as he set him down on a pillow, the kitty began to snooze.

Our kitchen wasn't exactly an ideal spot, I thought, but the Formica countertop would do in a pinch. After ten minutes, I asked my son to check on the cat—mainly because I liked the fact that he was showing so much interest. The other kids were ensconced in the living room watching a late-night horror movie. Knowing Sherry wouldn't approve, we all agreed never to tell her.

As I fetched my sedated patient and laid him gently on the towel, Karen gave me one of her disgusted looks and stalked off. Draping the cat's hindquarters with paper towels, and gingerly plucking the hair from his scrotal sac, I proceeded to extract the two, spherical testosterone-producing nodules. "Geeze, Don, he's built like a Brahma bull...but we're almost done." Turning pale, Don was obviously queasy. Quickly sitting down in the closest chair, he buried his head in his hands mumbling, "Just tell me when it's over."

But K.C. was fascinated, and I had to push his head away from my field of vision more than once. One quick suture, then another—and my night's work was done. The actual neutering had taken just a few minutes, and it was virtually bloodless.

Stroking the kitten's long black tail, I moved his sleeping body back into Don's box. "Now, take Sylvester and your kids home. Put the kitty in your small guest bedroom and close the door. Let him awaken slowly...and tell Sherry to not let him go outside for at least five nights, no matter how much he begs."

"Okay, thanks Uncle Doc. Kids, let's go home, Mama's waiting."

Karen happily closed and double-locked the door behind all three, while trying in vain to sound sincere, "Good night, hope to see y'all again real soon." She still couldn't believe I had castrated Sylvester on her kitchen counter. While I nonchalantly folded the towel and began to clean the area with the nearest sponge, she grabbed my arm. "Oh, no you don't! What are you thinking? That's what I use on our dishes. I give up...I just give up!"

"Sorry, but it's only a little kitty fuzz," I said as I quickly tossed the sponge back where I found it.

This time, her cheeks flushed when she yelled, "Now throw that away! This ain't the clinic. Good gosh, you went to medical school and were taught all about germs...but you end up putting that dirty sponge back into my clean sink?"

The whole scene was so bizarre that Karen couldn't help herself as she grinned and tried to stifle a laugh. She knew that, in order to move right along, I'd been conditioned to wipe up with the closest thing handy. It wasn't as though I'd done an autopsy. In fact, I'd made bigger messes cooking breakfast sausages. But it was too late. She was still shaking her head in dismay as she tried changing the subject, "When he wakes up, won't Sylvester be crying and howling all night long?"

As in the past, our laughing together always seemed to change any prevailing mood. "Yeah, but he won't be crying from pain. He'll be scratching at the door and hollering to go outside. I'd say that'll be more than enough to pay back Don and Sherry for wakin' us up."

Standing there, still holding Sylvester's tiny two organs in the palm of my hand, I opened the cabinet door below the sink to throw them out when K.C. squealed, "Oh, Dad...how gross!"

"Don't put those in my trash!" Karen ordered again. So I started to put them into the automatic disposal, instead. But before I could flip the switch, Karen cringed and shouted, "No! I can't believe you were going to do that...I can't stand it!"

"What?" I argued, "It's no worse than washing giblets down the drain."

"Yes, it *is* worse. If you had done that, every time I'd go to use the disposal again, I'd see Sylvester's face. Let's just go to bed...I don't even want to think about what you might do next."

Putting her arm around our son, Karen giggled to herself as the two of them sleepily made their way back down the darkened hallway to their bedrooms—hoping against hope to be able to fall asleep. It was now one o'clock in the morning.

Out of respect for Karen's feelings, as well as Sylvester's dignity…I carefully wrapped his manhood in double layers of foil and placed it in the freezer. Since I'd be getting up before anyone else, I'd have a chance to take the small package with me to the clinic before my unsuspecting wife and son knew anything. But this whole episode made me realize how little people want to know about what really goes on behind the scenes during and after any type of surgery, whether on humans or animals.

When I finally shuffled back to bed, Karen drowsily mumbled, "By the way, I've set the clock for five o'clock. I'm going to wake Sherry to tell her that you and K.C. will be at their place tomorrow night—at midnight—to pick up the extra symphony tickets Don said she had." I knew she was just kidding. But she did manage to get in one more jibe, "And, honey, before you hurt yourself, I think you should put K.C.'s plastic water gun back into his desk."

Though I remembered to put the fake pistol away, I forgot all about the foil package in the refrigerator. A couple of weeks later, when Karen asked me what it was, I nonchalantly told her it was just a lab sample that I'd be taking to the clinic. She didn't ask any more questions.

2

True Test

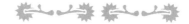

N o one clicked...even though we rushed to interview whomever we could, whenever we could. This was a real dilemma. In our excitement to settle into our spiffy Meadow Creek Clinic, we'd made the move too soon. With no additional staff, as well as leaving Twin Oaks without a new vet, I imagined a future of eighteen-hour days. It was impossible to think that just the four of us, two doctors and two assistants, could shuttle between both of these clinics forever. The applicants who were the right match had little experience, while others with experience insisted on more perks than we could deliver. The rest were simply turned off by our visibly tough workload, since we were still administering to horses, cattle and everything in between. Younger city vets wanted an easier lifestyle, caring for poodles and kittens, and we couldn't blame them.

Then along came Dr. Wm. Mathew Horton. Not only was he the spitting image of my partner, Dr. Rich Vest, but he also appeared just as capable and professional. Personable, too...I liked his approach. "Heard you been lookin' for help. I can do whatever needs to be done, whenever it needs doin'." Then looking at me straight on, he said, "Doc, what I don't know, I can learn. And what I haven't seen...*you* have." His comment, good-natured as it was, suddenly made me feel like a grizzled ol' timer.

Tall and slender with a head of thick brown hair, he must have appeared irresistible to women. Tracy and Rachelle nearly tripped over themselves to stare at him. And I was in awe. The fellow even came dressed for action, in a pressed green smock, starched Wrangler jeans, and polished, but worn, calfskin boots. Totally at ease with himself, work-coveralls were thrown over his shoulder, a thermometer stuck out of his left pocket, and his stethoscope was in hand. This was all too perfect, and I felt that Dr. Vest might be playing another one of his pranks. How could such a well-suited veterinarian just drop into our laps?

I didn't want to doubt this miracle. If it were a joke, I'd go along for the ride. I didn't intend to chitchat either, for fear he'd disappear in a puff of smoke. So I tossed the fellow right into the fray. "Matt, we'd like you to see our patient in exam room #3."

We both knew this was a test, of sorts. But I was the only one to tag along for his evaluation, since Dr. Vest would be out of action for a while with a broken leg. He'd been

chasing after a runaway goat at the McKinney ranch, and
took a flying spill over a broken rake. Using the phone next
to the exam room to check on his condition at the hospital, I
also listened in on Dr. Horton's diagnosis for the eye problem
our patient was having. The Shar-pei puppy, 'Chang', suffered
from entropion. I'd noticed his eyelid inversions during his
first visit for vaccinations, and recommended their correction.
But his owner, Corey Carole, hadn't returned. So Matt was
now seeing the chronic effects of how the excessive skin folds
in this breed were causing Chang's eyelashes to rub against
his eyeballs. Trying to peer out through swollen slits, the little
blond pup squinted from the aggravated tearing. In pain and
irritable, he ducked his head away from any attempts to pet
him on the brow. "He acts like he's blind," whined Corey.

Speaking softly, Dr. Horton simply said, "You're
partially right."

After leaving a message for Rich, I stood in the
background while Dr. Horton continued his exam. Corey, an
extroverted college freshman with kinky blond curls, was as
cute as her pup, but surprisingly contrary to suggestions or
advice. Matt didn't beat around the bush. Firmly expressing
disappointment that she'd waited so long, he described the
corrective surgical procedure urgently needed for Chang. The
argumentative young lady had no choice but to agree.

Though Matt had just met our ace staff, it seemed as
though he'd worked with them for years. "Okay, Tracy, let's
move... ain't no time like the present," he said as he hurriedly

scooped Chang up into his arms and rushed by me to the surgical suite.

"Right now?" asked our incredulous assistant.

"Ain't no sense in wastin' good daylight," Dr. Horton said. This was, indeed, a man after my own heart.

When Chang was anesthetized, I contentedly leaned against the wall and observed Dr. Horton's steady hands and flawless technique as he performed the delicate face-lift. Elliptical incisions above and below the eyes allowed the eyelashes to turn outward. He sewed in a difficult averting pattern. During the procedure, I said nothing and offered no coaching. After Matt tied the last stitch, I had to ask the question: "How many of these particular surgeries have you done?"

"One," he answered.

* * * * *

My partner hobbled into work a few days later. Wearing a pair of oversized, striped black and white overalls to hide his full leg cast, Rich looked like a stick in a barrel.

"Wish I'd been here...how did y'all get everything done?"

"Matt and I worked both clinics, but I'm not rightly sure how we did it. We were movin' so fast, our shadows seldom crossed." I'd already told him earlier how lucky we were this fellow came along, but nothing could be final until he agreed with me.

Rich kept peeking down the hallway like he was on some spy mission. "...and what in the devil are you looking for?" I asked.

"The whiz of a new vet," he said. "It's bad enough I had to break my leg before you hired us some help, but now you've probably gone and run 'im off already."

"You limped right past him...he's standing in the waiting room with Mel Crosby," I explained, realizing Rich was feeling strange about this new development.

"*That* young fella out there...naw, couldn't be."

"Hell," I laughed. "...you were young lookin' once, too. But I haven't hired him yet. Like I said, that'll be up to you."

I followed Dr. Vest's lopsided walk to the front desk, and made introductions all around. Rising to the occasion, Rich became his usual jovial self, teasing Matt about the necessity of getting out on the road and meeting some of the local color.

Mel, our busiest rancher, anxiously interrupted, "Yeah, let's go Docs...c'mon...I've got a cow waitin' that's in sad shape with a prolapsed uterus and one of my horses got somethin' in his eye."

In Italian loafers with tassels, Mel Crosby didn't fit the image of a big Texas ranch owner. And I always wondered why he never wore a hat, since there was a perennial shiny glaze on his sunburned bald spot. Though a mite short, when he stood erect he gave the impression of being tall and austere until you shook his hand. Then you knew immediately he was as down to earth as a fence post. His strong grip felt like no

other. And in the scratchiness of his voice, it was easy to hear
something sincere and honest. A real Texan.

We followed Mel's truck out to the rolling hills of his
Preston Bend spread, bordering the high lands between the
east and west forks of the Trinity River. As a history buff, I
was always spouting off facts about our area. And I tried to
impress Matt by telling him that the founder of Dallas, John
Neely Bryan, used the very same trail in 1841 to trade pelts
and hides with the Caddo Indians. And this was before the
Three Forks battle that eventually led to the settlement of the
territory. Rich suddenly groaned, but not because he'd heard
this dozens of times before. He winced with pain, grabbing
his leg to keep it steady as my truck rumbled and rocked
through a muddy wash.

We stopped by the impressive stone house built by his
great-grandfather, and Mel quickly changed clothes. Then
leading us past a meadow of wild yellow daffodils, he took
us to the pasture where his herd of more than a hundred
Quarter horse mares was grazing. Pointing toward a cluster of
pipe corrals next to the river's bend, he said, "Docs, Tom and
Kirby will bring Spot and her calf down to those pens." And
he hollered over to his two hands to ride. Already saddled,
the nodding cowboys, who couldn't have been more than
eighteen, went galloping into the sun seemingly confident of
finding the shorthorn cow.

"This could take forever," Matt whispered.

Ten minutes went by. Then Mel used his truck's horn
to blare out three long blasts. Waiting another five minutes,

he again blasted three more honks. A low *moo-oo* sound was heard in the east. Suddenly Tom came thundering along the river's edge with Spot and her calf trying to run ahead of both horse and rider. Whooping and hollering, "Git up ther', Spot," he managed to maneuver both into the pens, but the half-hungry calf kept squalling long after the gates were slammed behind them.

I'd never known a rancher to train herds in this way. And it was a sight to see. Conditioned to the sound of Mel's horn, along the ridge appeared two thousand or more head of cattle answering his call. Matt gasped, "Just how many do you graze?"

Waving to Kirby as the lad came loping out from the brush, Mel laughed, "One too many...especially when it comes to paying feed and vet bills."

After climbing between the metal bars of the fence, Dr. Horton and I examined the ailing cow. As the calf tried in vain to suckle milk from her udder, I circled to the right and Matt moved around to the left of Spot's horns. It was obvious why Mel called her Spot. She was a brown and black brindle with a solid white patch of fur in the center of her back. But she spooked when Matt and I came around to her backside. "Dern it," he sighed heavily when he saw what I'd just seen. Spot's condition was far worse than any of us could have expected.

After delivering a healthy heifer, most of her reproductive tract was now turned inside out. The largest portion of her hemorrhagic uterus was dragging on the ground behind her hocks. It looked like some sort of purple and battered, forty-pound 'thing' trying to come out from the depths of her bowels. Leaves and dirt coated the bloody mucus lining that left a slimy trail in the sand...attracting flies.

"When did this cow prolapse?" asked Matt.

"This mornin', I think," Mel said.

Kirby piped up, "Maybe yesterday..."

"No, mighta been longer," added Tom.

I shrugged and looked at Dr. Vest, while we waited for Dr. Horton to speak. We both felt this was Matt's case. It wasn't so much what he said, but how he spoke to our rancher client. This would determine if Mel would accept the young vet's recommendations. I walked away, and waited.

"Well...can you help 'er?" asked the rancher as he turned to Matt.

"Her breedin' days are over, but I can maybe keep her alive to nurse that baby."

"How?" Mel asked.

"By cuttin' that mess off," Matt answered.

"Hmm, no fancy words, boy?" Mel challenged Matt as he reached in his pocket for a fresh chaw of tobacco.

"Nope," Matt said, while tearing a pinch from the plug that Mel offered.

"How much will it cost me?"

"Less money than she's worth dead," Matt retorted.

"Could she die?" chimed in Tom.

"Well...she damn sure can't stay the way she is," Matt answered.

With a Texas rancher, sometimes saying less was better than saying more. Stroking his chin and shuffling in his boots, Mel was thinking. "Well..." he finally said, looking Matt up and down, "...have you ever done one of these?"

"Nope," was the immediate reply.

I liked the answer—direct and honest. He didn't apologize or shun the responsibility. I was amazed at his grit and natural instincts. Though originally from Utah, his previous experience had been limited to city clinics. While I wondered what the cattleman would say next, Dr. Vest spoke up. "Mel, give 'im a chance. And while Dr. Horton fixes your cow, I'll take a look at your horse's eye."

"Do whatcha gotta do, Docs," Mel said, as he motioned for Rich to follow him. The rancher climbed through the fence and walked toward the corral. "I'll tell ya, Doc, found that mare late last night. It was her right eye. Musta poked it on somethin'." He looked over his shoulder to watch Dr. Horton prepare to work on Spot, while I helped gather the medicines and instruments needed. Turning back to Rich, he added, "Well, anyway...I packed it with salt."

"You did what?" Dr. Vest asked with alarm.

Matt was in the middle of rolling a pair of plastic-glove obstetrical sleeves up to his shoulders when we both overheard the remarks and shuddered.

This was a side of Mel we'd never seen, and it concerned us, especially when he added, " Yeah, I've come to find that if salt doesn't blind 'em...then, they'll be a purdy good horse."

Rich was visibly disturbed, "Mel, haven't you ever heard of eye ointments?"

"Dr. V...have you ever tried to put ointment in a wild bronc's eye?" asked Kirby, coming to the defense of his boss.

"Besides," Tom added, "after that salt treatment, whenever Mr. Crosby yells 'Whoa'...I'll betcha that horse stops on a dime." I suppose each man reckoned he had a point, but it would be something we'd be discouraging from here on out. In fact, we urged the boys to call us first before anyone on the ranch resorted to that outdated and dangerous treatment again.

Dr. Horton administered an epidural injection between the spinal vertebrae and Spot's loin to ensure restraint and relief from pain. And he gave her enough lidocaine to deaden her hindquarters, but keep her standing.

Deciding to wait before seeing the mare, Mel and Dr. Vest couldn't resist coming back to observe Dr. Horton's heroic attempt to save Spot. While Matt straddled the cow's engorged uterus, I held her tail away from his face. "Please don't fall on me," he mumbled to the cow, after assuring himself there was no bladder damage.

Matt felt he had to let us know each and every step he made: "Docs, I'm going to infiltrate the base of the organ with local anesthetic. Then to shrink the vascular vessels, I'll inject epinephrine and place large sutures to seal the uterine stump before replacing it back into the vaginal area. Then, I'll be suturing her vulva to hold everything in place."

Talking it through seemed to make him and Mel feel better. But Dr. Vest and I knew it wasn't going to be simple. All his intentions were medically sound, but realistically futile. Matt scrubbed and disinfected the area. As soon as he perforated the raw tissues with the large ligature needle, blood shot clear across his shoulder. With the second attempt, his face and chest were showered and Spot swung her rump around. Though she felt no pain, her hooves stirred up mounds of fire ants just before she urinated down the front of Matt's coveralls. I jumped on the fence, and Dr. Vest ran to the horse trough to soak ants away from his boots and pant-cuffs.

"Well, let's try that again," Matt calmly said, "...and bring her down here to the trough." I admired his guts, and led Spot to the end of the water trough.

Standing knee-deep in water, Matt asked Mel to tie Spot's horns to the post, while I was to hold her tail through the fence. "I'll let her uterus float in this trough until I finish what I started."

Surgical gloves flew off and blood vessels spurted, but Matt continued to suture, until ten knots were tied and the uterine body was cut off. When the cervical stump stopped oozing, the determined newcomer sighed, "Now, we can put it back inside and complete the suturing."

In unison, Mel and the boys asked if Spot would be okay. And Dr. Vest chimed in, "She'll be fit as a fiddle. And,

hey, Natty...that was a damn fine job." Oddly enough, the
offhanded nickname stuck.

"Natty," Mel repeated, " I'd be obliged if you'd take a
look at my bay mare's eye now...since Dr. Vest hasn't seen her
yet." There it was, I thought to myself—the rancher's stamp
of approval.

Matt sloshed out from the trough with his jeans
sagging to the ground, and walked over to the broodmare
brought in by Kirby. Rank and pasture bred, an old fight
scar could be seen on one side of her neck and a fresh cut
appeared above her nostril. Mel called her 'Witch', but
'Bewitched' suited her better. Irritably pawing, she struck at
Dr. Horton twice, and even tried to bite Kirby. But as soon as
Mel whispered, "Whoa," the horse stood perfectly still. And
her eye looked normal—clear as could be.

With his hand on Matt's shoulder, the cattleman asked,
"Well, Doc....?

"Mr. Crosby, sir," Matt said, "I'd say...she looks fine
and must be a purdy good horse."

"I reckon we're all through here now, so let's roll,"
my partner said as he got into Ol' Blue and hunkered down
in the seat. I figured he must be worn out since this was his
first day of getting around on his cast. I wondered if he liked
Matt, and why he'd chosen to give him a nickname. After
all, 'Natty' and 'Matty' were pretty much the same. But I
chalked it up to just another one of Rich's eccentricities. I did
think, though, that it might have been because Matt was so
persistent about everything, like a gnat. But I suppose that

odd association was just one of *my* eccentricities. Whatever the reason...his name remained 'Natty' from then on.

The dome light flickered when we crawled inside the cab. It must have been a sight to see, three bedraggled, tired and dirty vets sitting shoulder to shoulder in silence. The only sound was the dripping from Matt's pant-cuffs onto the floorboard. I was about to start the engine when Dr. Vest broke the silence, "Natty...would you like a fulltime job?"

Grinning widely, and in a voice barely above a whisper, the young man said, "Nope, got one...working with y'all."

Nothing else needed to be said.

3

Unforgettable Lessons

R achel, usually unflappable, was verbally stumbling again over the change in phone announcements. It was 12:02 when she answered our line with her usual upbeat "Twin Oaks...I mean Meadow Creek Animal Clinic, Good Morning." Whoever was on the line began correcting her...making our receptionist even more tongue-tied. "Yes, Ma'am. No, ma'am, you're right...it's not...it should be 'Good Afternoon.'"

I didn't know anyone who would bother to fuss so about a two minute difference. Though one person could qualify: my former grade school teacher, Nita Crow. Mrs.Crow took great joy in having you repeat whatever verbal lesson she had in mind for you. English was her subject and her life; a life made all the more difficult by having to teach the children of Texas. These were kids who would never take a shine to her need for both perfect grammar and precise punctuality.

I enjoyed pulling her leg, though. So when Rachel nodded to me that it was indeed Mrs. Crow, I spoke loud enough for Nita to hear me. "Gimme *tha* talk box." Then taking the phone, I continued speaking like a country bumpkin, thinking I'd get a laugh out of her. "Whatcha doin', gal? I ain't seen ya of late. How ya been gittin' around, and where's that sorry man-eatin' dog *a yurs*, Charlie?"

"That is the very reason I'm calling today. The yearly rabies vaccination for my Dalmatian is now due." Her clear diction was that of an Oxford graduate. My hands went clammy and my shoulders cramped in anxiety, just like they did when I sat in her classroom. I knew better, of course, but the old conditioning took over whenever I heard her voice.

Mrs. Crow's canine had an infamous reputation for having a cranky attitude. Vets and mailmen were at the top of his hate list. Charlie had laid into Ned Gilmore, the postal carrier in Nita's neighborhood, biting him four times. Though the wounds weren't serious, Mrs. Crow still ran the risk of losing her dog unless she erected a fence separating Charlie from the post-drop box.

In Nita's eyes, Charlie was the dog-of-dogs, and he, in turn, worshipped her. But, for many reasons, Nita knew it would be best not to come into our clinic anymore. After digging Charlie's snarling teeth out from the yoke of his boot, Dr. Vest swore never to touch him again. And one of Tracy's uniform sleeves still bears a snag after he snapped at her when we first began treating him for a lung disease.

"Dr. Carlton, may I make an appointment for Charlie here at my home?" asked the school marm.

"Yes, you can." I said.

In her serious tone, she said, "No, no...Yes, you *may*."

Ribbing her more, I added, "Limme see, if it don't rain and the crick don't rise, I'll be there in a bit."

Enjoying the game, she quipped, "Dr. Carlton, exactly how long is a bit?"

I could already see her standing there with her left hand on her hip, and a slight frown across her brow.

After responding with, "Ma'am, a bit is just one letter short of a bite, and almost longer than a while," I figured that might bring an end to our sparring for the day.

So far, I'd been the only one Charlie hadn't chomped on. I knew his disposition wasn't his entire fault. He had serious issues that were only compounded by the local school kids who continuously teased him through the cyclone fence on their way home. So the poor dog became tense and ready for action as soon as he heard the ringing of the afternoon school bell. Since the students couldn't take their anger out on Mrs. Crow, Charlie ended up taking the 'rap' for her stern, unforgiving discipline in the classroom.

"How's 'bout two o'clock?" I slurred, knowing I'd be late. "Whaddya *thank?*"

Feigning a dramatic southern accent, Nita said, "I think, sir, that you are taking liberties with me. But I will certainly expect you to be prompt."

I had to admire Nita's constant care for her difficult pet. And truth be told, I liked Charlie, too. He'd had tough times to overcome, and his valiant spirit never yielded. As a pup, he had a mamma as mean as a one-eyed bobcat and his papa fought off packs of stray dogs roaming the junkyard. But things only got worse for this critter.

Nita first brought Charlie in to us because he was severely underweight and coughing constantly. He also had persistent diarrhea. Our radiographs showed irregular nodules in his chest and liver, and a gross enlargement of his spleen. The anemia and high fever, coupled with the fact that he slept under the chicken coop didn't help any. Numerous blood profiles and a bone marrow biopsy were drawn to confirm our diagnosis of the chronic condition. The Dalmatian had 'histoplasmosis', an air-borne fungal disease that attacks the lungs. The extensive treatments were no walk-in-the-park for Charlie. The multiple, daily ketoconazole injections, and continual lab testing took their toll, making him more irritable than ever. He'd been sickly for so long and had spent so many miserable days in the hospital before recovering, that I offered to make only house calls whenever he needed care.

Tracy and I pulled into Mrs. Crow's driveway around three o'clock. Since Ol' Blue's wheels didn't fit onto the two concrete strips leading back to the garage, we burned rubber

and clattered along—the sound of which got Charlie to
barking furiously. Tracy was apprehensive, but I noted that
maybe he'd changed some now that he was healthy again.

We were sure Nita's house looked darn near as it did a
hundred years ago. It appeared solid enough, though, since it
was built during the time when red rock walls were customary
and tall gabled framing was the classic architectural choice. I
assumed she had the same lace window curtains behind her
perennially closed, brown shutters. The lamp on her porch
was lit both day and night, but I didn't believe anyone had
ever been through the archway of the front door. This was a
solitary woman with few friends and no family that I knew
of. Now that she was retired, I wondered why she didn't
occasionally enjoy the company of her former colleagues.
She'd taught at the same school, just a block from her home,
for nearly forty years.

We stopped near the side door leading to the kitchen.
Just a few steps marked the entryway, but they were so badly
decayed that the edges had crumbled away completely. This
could be dangerous for the heavy-set woman. So Tracy and I
considered sending someone out to repair the stairs for her.
We did notice, though, the old fence separating this entrance
and Charlie's backyard had been replaced with a brand new
one. And signs of fresh cement patching were evident along
the walkway.

Nita's shadow appeared behind the warped screen door
just as she kicked at the base frame to open it. As she stepped
out, the old door squeaked and slammed behind her.

"If looks could kill," whispered Tracy.

"I've been waiting and waiting," Nita scolded. "And I told Charlie you would probably be late—as usual."

Old habits die hard, and, 'as usual', I tried to avoid eye contact with Mrs. Crow.

Charlie sat patiently behind the new chain-link fence, but his tail was rigged and he looked none too happy to see me. It was obvious that he'd gained around thirty pounds. This was a good sign. And his black spots were now stretched and taut. Gone was the former emaciated look of dehydration.

It was after we stepped inside that I saw how much Nita had changed during the past months. She seemed years older. Her haunting expression hadn't changed, and was even more exaggerated by wrinkles. The aging of her face only seemed to accentuate the glare I'd seen a thousand times. I always felt she could have been the original model for the often-repeated line, "That teacher has eyes in the back of her head."

Her hair, now gray, was still kept in a tight bun, and her black orthopedic shoes were laced to perfection. There was something here, though, that didn't fit the grimness: color. Nita's love of flowers and color showed up everywhere. Her kitchen seemed to vibrate in bright greens, yellows and pinks, betraying a passionate side of her that I never fully appreciated. Until now, I'd never seen her in anything other than a blue or black suit. But she was quite the sight in her loose-fitting sunflower dress, with a contrasting floral patterned apron tied in a bow at her waist. Even the porcelain mixing-bowl in her hands was green and orange.

As she turned to set the bowl down on the chrome-legged Formica table, I said, "I'll bet Charlie ain't none too happy about waiting, neither."

My former instructor snapped, ""Please, doctor...you know better than to use a double negative in a sentence."

"I didn't, I used a triple," I answered in a sassy tone which I immediately regretted...telling myself that I wasn't a ten-year-old anymore. Despite the fact that she often brought out the worst in me, I reminded myself that I needed to grow up and start acting professionally.

Tracy reviewed our simple plan of action: Nita would slip the restraining loop of our catchpole-snare around Charlie's neck to hold him briefly, while I popped him in the rear twice with the shots.

This time, Nita used her hip to push open the screen door. But Charlie heard it and knew we were coming. He tucked in his tail and ran to his favorite hiding spot. He knew better than try to oppose his mistress.

His dark eyes peeped out from under the floorboards of the abandoned chicken coop, which hadn't been used since his illness. These days, Charlie slept in the super-sized, warm doghouse that Nita had built for him. And he only retreated to the coop when he was frightened. We could see him crouching and huddling beneath the wood slats. So Nita crawled on her hands and knees around the edge, waiting for a chance to grab him. But whenever she got near enough to poke the pole at his nose or rear, he dodged her—again and again.

It was 110 degrees in the sun, and Nita perspired with exasperation. She went from gentle coaxing to anger, "Charlie, you old hound, you ain't worth all this."

Tracy and I looked at one another in astonishment. And my assistant couldn't resist, "*Isn't* worth all this."

But it wasn't the time or place for word games. I told Nita to stop trying so hard...that I may have a way of getting him out. At least I thought I did.

Fetching my lariat from Ol' Blue, I darted to the front of the house and hung my lasso over the fence. When the closing bells from the elementary school began to ring, I started prancing up and down on the outside of the fence, teasing the way the kids did. I rapped on the gate with a small stick and shook at the latch. Then I threw a handful of gravel at the side of the woodshed. From what I remembered, this is what usually made Charlie race toward the fence in anger.

But nothing happened. Tracy whistled and hooted. And behaving like a crazy school boy, I began singing like his hecklers, "You can't get me...you can't get me." But Charlie must have been bright enough to know this was a charade. He didn't budge.

Another thought came to mind when I saw Ned, the mailman, turn the corner at the end of the block. Running to meet him and quickly setting up a plan, I put on his jacket and hat, grabbed his mail pouch, and made my way toward the front of the house with my back turned. This image of a postman's rear proved too irresistible for Charlie and he shot out from beneath the coop at full speed toward the fence, locking his fangs into the steel webbing. I immediately turned and dropped the loop of my rope over his head before he could race back under the shed.

Nita tied him to the clothesline pole and Tracy used the snare of the catchpole as a muzzle.

"I can hold him still," Nita said, as she tried straddling Charlie's back, her ample buttocks high in the air. Dalmatians are tall animals, so it wasn't easy. And it was a sight I'll not soon forget. But I hoped I wouldn't end up giving her the shots. Nita grabbed Charlie by the ears, and clamped her knees tight against his ribs...like she was jockey on a racehorse. "Quickly, Doctor, give him the shots right now!" Charlie didn't flinch. And when we let him go, he stood there docilely as Nita stroked his head and praised him.

In the sun, I could see that Nita's weathered face was more like that of a farmer, since she probably spent countless hours in her garden. When I asked why she thought Charlie didn't respond to our pretense at being school kids, she said, "It may have taken me a while, but I finally realized that neither Charlie nor I needed to live with verbal abuse any longer. We're two of a kind. So, now, whenever the school bell goes off, I bring him inside with me. He gets a treat and I have my afternoon tea. Charlie's a smart dog, you know. And it delights me that I now have more time to spend with him."

After thanking us profusely, my former school teacher walked back to her kitchen, with Charlie next to her—looking every inch the handsome breed that he was as he strutted on inside. No matter how you looked at it, that tough dog and that stubborn woman were courageous forces to be reckoned with. And I came away with nothing but respect for the two of them.

4

Poker and Pranks

As fierce dust-devil storms whipped in from west Texas, power throughout most of Dallas shut down. Murky red clouds churned through the skies, and dry winds blew in a bone-numbing cold. With no electricity or phone service, Meadow Creek clinic would need to shut down for the day—not the best omen for our new beginning.

During this extreme weather, very few people would attempt to venture away from their homes. Dozens of repair crews branched out in response to the urgent need to get the metropolis up and running as swiftly as possible. And their trucks could be seen everywhere as they scrambled to fix downed trees, poles and twisted wires.

"What'll we do now?" asked Tracy, "At least all the animals in our wards have been treated and are doing well, but I'm worried about any that might be out there caught in the storm."

All I could think of was relishing a few peaceful hours, with the afternoon off. Dr. Vest was over at the other clinic helping out Dr. Horton and Rachel since Twin Oaks still had power. But here at Meadow Creek, my softhearted technician and Frank, our new kennel boy, were suddenly sitting idle; something neither one was accustomed to.

"Let's lock up for the afternoon, but I'll call you if we have an emergency," I said, though I had a secret plan of my own on how to utilize the rest of the day.

When my wife called to let me know utilities at her tack shop were still on, I headed Ol' Blue in her direction just a few miles away.

Karen was packing up saddles and bits for an upcoming horse show in Ft. Worth, and was in an especially good mood when I got there. My timing was perfect, "Honey, would y'all mind if me and the boys played a game of poker today?"

We needed a place to play, and her store was as inviting a spot as any. With its designed aisles of dry goods for horses and riders, green carpeting, Mexican floor tiles, and mahogany walls...the ambience was perfect. I loved this place; it was a horseman's dream. Track lights lit up display cases of turquoise jewelry, exotic boot skins, silver buckles, spurs, bits and hand-tooled leathers of crafted saddle pommels and stirrups. Not a single currycomb or harness was out of place.

But she didn't volunteer her shop. So I watched her work and drove her crazy by following her around like a lost puppy. I kept begging to use her back room for our game. As she moved past the riding helmets, brushes and leg wraps, and reached up to dust the short cantle of an English saddle, she continued to be unresponsive. Finally, unable to stand me at her heels, she relented, "Okay, but only on two conditions. If you promise that my store won't smell like cigar smoke afterwards...and if you'll keep the doors open for customers until closing time."

"Deal," I agreed, and dashed to the counter to make quick calls to four buddies whom I rarely had the chance to see anymore. With most of Dallas shut down, no one refused. At three o'clock, just as my pals began arriving, Karen took off. But as she got in the car, she couldn't resist wagging her finger at me, "Y'all better be good, and mind the store."

As though he'd been waiting for the call, Dr. Laurel Buford, a pathologist at St. Luke's Hospital, brought the cards. After commenting that the tack shop was as immaculate as any surgical suite, he began arranging our game table in the back room next to the alley. Cyrus Clark, a local chiropractor who always dressed in army fatigues, pushed the alley door open for air, as he fired up the butt-end of his smoke-billowing Cuban cigar. And Dr. Danny Zeff, a pediatric specialist still in surgical scrubs, rocked contentedly in his chair stuffing himself with molasses-flavored leaves of chewing tobacco—something his wife forbade him to do at home. I was sure I could find a spittoon cup for him somewhere amongst Karen's sale items. While I searched, Dr. Ty 'Red' Mason rushed in...the last to arrive. A gynecologist with Dallas General, and the youngest of our group, Red just got out of surgery. Smiling broadly, he cozied up to the round table and cut the deck. These guys were ready for business.

I couldn't help but think that the combined medical experience of these gents hunkered around the card table was at least a hundred and forty years. Then Cyrus leaned back in the metal folding chair, flicking an ash on the vinyl floor, and hollered, "Hey, Doc, come on...we're ready to deal."

Feeling somewhat guilty as I turned the front door sign over to CLOSED, I eagerly skipped to the back of the store. In this stock room of boot boxes and racks of woven reins the air was pungent with the smell of leather, and just right for the nice little gambling den we'd fashioned out for ourselves. Popping open the lid of his ice chest, Red cheerily asked, "Beer or pretzels?" Despite the short notice, this fellow had come prepared.

As Danny took a swig of whisky from his handy silver flask, he offered it to Laurel, razzing him, "Here, try this stuff. It'll put hair on that bald dome of yours."

I sat between the two, while Red dealt the first hand.

Suddenly everyone spoke at once, "Doc...there's the doorbell. Thought you closed up."

"I did...."

"Anyone in here?" shouted a voice from out front.

Pushing away from the table, I grumbled, "Splendid, just splendid. I'll be right back." For the first time since I

can't remember when, I'd been dealt a full house. I reluctantly
laid the cards face down, leaving behind the wisecracking
physicians, and walked out to greet the unwelcome customer.
"Howdy, mister," I smiled, "I'm sorry, but we're closed." I
probably looked a little strange to him. My hat was snubbed
tight against the top of my ears and my denim pant legs were
scrunched up around the heels of my boots and spur rowels,
since my alternate plan was to ride my horse if the guys didn't
want to play cards.

"I'm Colonel Timothy A. Fairchild," the man said
in a haughty manner. It was apparent that he felt this
announcement would be important to me. I wondered why
he'd just walked in, paying no mind to the CLOSED sign.
Apparently I'd forgotten to lock the door with the deadbolt.
I wasn't impressed with his title, and his presence was already
grating on my nerves. Though taller than me, he was so
slump-shouldered that we faced eye to eye. Wearing high-
water jeans tucked inside the yokes of cheap, pointed-toed
cowboy boots, it was obvious he wasn't from these parts.
His bronze-plated belt buckle was partially hidden by the
overhang of his belly.

"Son, I need a blanket for my horse...and I'm in a
hurry," he demanded.

I dismissed the 'son' remark, and offered him an
ashtray since he was dropping cigarette ashes on Karen's
carpet. Again, I said, "I'm sorry, sir, but the store is closed.
If you'll come back tomorrow, I'm sure we'll be able to
help you."

"No, absolutely not. I want a blanket now, yee all."
His *yankeeness* was obscene. And I remembered something my
Uncle Grump always said about *damn* and *yankee* not being
separate words. In the colonel's case, *damnyankee* was one
word. His accent, rudeness and clothing gave him away. And
I reckoned he must have meant y'all, rather than *yee all*. We'd
had a recent influx of snow bunnies, and spotting them was a
little too easy.

I sensed that my buddies were listening at the back
door. But for Karen's sake, I was determined to show the
colonel some southern hospitality. Pointing to the rack where
winter horse blankets and hoods were displayed, I kindly
said, "We have those in stock, and more are available in the
storeroom."

"Not that kind of blanket, you fool...I want a blanket
for my horse's back."

Muffled snickers could be heard coming from the
storage room. "Perhaps a saddle pad, then?" I asked knowing
Karen had dozens of different styles near the front window,
ranging in price from $25 to $150.

His blood pressure must have been off the charts,
because his face was turning red with frustration. "Yes, a pad...
and would you hurry it up."

Smiling and nodding, I led Colonel Fairchild to
the stacks to make his choice. Grumbling to himself as he
rummaged through the inventory, he let every other pad drop
on the floor without putting any of them back. Then stepping
over the pile, said, "You can pick those up later...after all,

that's your job." He'd gone through two-dozen styles, and ten colors of each style—but none suited his fancy. "Is this all you have, is it?" As he became more brusque, it was all I could do to hold my tongue. When he snarled, "Look...I want the best. Money's no object. But if you don't hurry it up, I'm going to report you to the owner." Then under his breath, he slowly grunted, "Damn Texans."

Enough was enough. Cordially asking him to wait a moment, I wheeled around and flew into the storeroom. My friends sat there quietly scowling, with their arms folded tightly across their chests.

They were madder than hell. They'd heard the colonel, and didn't take well to his comment about Texans.

Poker became a thing of the past as the four medics plotted out a scheme to teach the *damnyankee* a lesson.

"Doc, take him this $250 pad," Cyrus directed.

"But that's from the $25 stack, I said.

Cyrus heels clicked together, "Yeah, but he's on our side of the Red River!"

Each doctor was a native Texan whom I'd known since grade school. We all shared strong chauvinistic feelings about our homestate. And the colonel had pushed all the wrong buttons.

Dutifully playing my part, I carried one blanket at a time from the room for the gentleman's inspection, as my four friends waited. Each time I walked through the door, one of them had the next newly priced saddle pad to be shown to the colonel. Of course, he'd already seen most of them out front, but didn't know the difference.

With devious calculation, the medics giddily continued marking new sales tags—getting bolder and bolder as time went on. Out of the corner of his mouth, Danny said, "Doc, now treat 'im like the *Good Book* says."

"Oh, I will," I said as I trotted out front with three more saddle pads, originally $100. Each was the same, except for the color. But the blue one was now $300, the white pad was $375, and the green one was $400. I spread them out over the display cases under different lighting. The brighter the light, the higher the price. But the colonel still wasn't finding what he wanted.

When Rachel called from Twin Oaks, I spoke loudly enough for the colonel to hear. "I'll need to call you back, I'm waiting on a very important customer."

"Sir, I have one really expensive pad that..." Hesitating a moment, I continued, "...but it's probably more than you'd ever want to spend."

"Son, it's about time you started showing me the good stuff."

Returning to the den of iniquity, I pulled out the bottom pad in the last stack, as Laurel dusted it off. It was a black, crushed-velvet Navaho pad with silver fringe. I remembered when Karen ordered it as a gift, because it looked good in the catalog's color photograph. But she hadn't been able to sell it or give it away. It was that bad.

"Gawd, that has to be the gaudiest thing I've ever seen," said Red.

Making a face, Cyrus mumbled, "Geeze, Doc, that's one ugly horse pad. I wouldn't even use it to line the trunk of my car."

Danny grinned, "Yeah, this is the one...that guy out there will think it's better than sex."

Grabbing my shoulder, Laurel whispered in my ear, "Doc, please let me make this sale."

Going back out front, I said, "Sir, I need to make a call, but this gentlemen will help you. He's our resident Chief of Staff."

Proudly holding the fringed pad in front of him, Laurel was enthusiastic, "Yes, Colonel Fairchild, this is the finest pad in the store. We ordered it special." He wasn't lying. It had been ordered, and it was in a special stack marked with Karen's handwritten note: 'Donate to Salvation Army'.

As I dialed Twin Oaks, I watched Laurel making the final pitch. For once, the colonel looked pleased.

Dr. Vest came on the line, but he wasn't laughing. "Doc, I've got a dog here you need to see."

"I'm kinda in the middle of something. Can't it wait?"

"No, it really can't."

Leaving by the alley door, I asked the boys to save my cards. "I'll try to be right back. And Red, help Buford with that sale."

When I got to the back entrance of Twin Oaks, Dr. Vest met me, "Doc, I haven't got a clue on how to handle this client."

Quickly removing my spurs, and putting on a smock, I asked what was wrong.

Shrugging his shoulders, Dr. Horton added, "The lady's name is Mirabelle Henderson...and nothin's wrong."

Sighing, Rich said, "Natty means there's nothing wrong with her dog, Scarlet. She's convinced that the corgi needs emergency surgery."

"And you called me into the clinic for no reason?"

"You've got to see this for yourself," they said. "She's insistent."

The mystery of all this piqued my curiosity. And sure enough, there was Mirabelle standing in the exam room, clutching her small white and brown corgi like it might be the last time she'd ever see her alive.

The woman was near tears when she spoke. I couldn't make out her long, slow drawl, and figured she might be from Mississippi. While we talked, Scarlet squirmed out of her grasp and Mirabelle let her play on the floor. The pup seemed normal and peppy. But her owner was certain something was wrong.

Both Rich and Natty stayed in the room with me when I gave the pooch another thorough checkup. Her eyes, ears, heart and lungs were fine. She had no abdominal discomfort, and no unusual discharges or sounds. And nothing seemed broken or sprained. In fact, Scarlet was enjoying the attention, and her tongue was wagging as fast as her nubbed tail.

"She appears healthy, ma'am...what makes you think she needs surgery?" I asked.

"I was told she did," the pretty brunette answered as she hugged Scarlet close.

Dr. Horton interjected, "By whom?"

"By my groomer," Mrs. Henderson replied.

Not wanting to rush to judgment, I merely repeated, "Your groomer? And why did she come to that conclusion?"

"She said there was an...odor."

"An odor?" we all echoed together.

"Yes, sir...she said Scarlet's kidneys were bad, and she'd need a $2,000 operation."

Now I was really taken aback, and wondered if her groomer was performing illegal kidney transplants. In fact, in all my years in veterinary medicine, I've never even performed such a transplant.

This was an astonishing development, and more than a little worrisome. I examined Scarlet again, but there were no signs of a vaginal or anal gland discharge, and her temperature was normal. There was also no unusual odor. We all sniffed her while she licked my hand. We even smelled her breath. Nothing. The pup's teeth were spotless, and her gums were pink. We were bewildered, but continued searching for anything we might have missed.

"Does she drink a lot of water?" Dr. Vest asked when he inquired if the dog had ever shown signs of illness.

And Dr. Horton asked if the dog had been spayed, or if there'd ever been signs of blood in her urine or stool.

After reviewing all the facts again, I said, "So what we have here is a groomer's diagnosis. Will you excuse our medical team for a moment, Miss Henderson, while we confer on this case?"

As soon as we closed the door behind us, Rich rolled his eyes, "Now can you see why we've been so confused? "

I stood there dumfounded, trying to put the pieces together. I suppose it was possible that Scarlet may have a bladder or kidney infection, but she sure didn't need a transplant. Something was very wrong here, but we couldn't ignore the complaint. I also wanted to get the name of her groomer and do a bit of investigation.

Dr. Horton had been talking quietly to Tracy in the pharmacy area, so I called him over to discuss my decision. "Doctors, " I said, "we can't rule out anything, so let's run a CBC and blood chemistry profile to check on the dog's cell counts and organ functions. Then we can follow up with a urinalysis and pneumocystogram. I'd also like to see a urine cytology prior to the urethral catheterization and pneumatic dilation of her bladder for radiographs."

Looking straight at Dr. Horton, I added, "Or...we can do nothing...and just watch you squirm while we pile up all these expensive tests." Dr. Vest tried to keep a straight face, but Natty blushed when I shouted, "Gotcha! You can tell your actress, Mirabelle, that her accent isn't real and it helped to give her away."

Rachel sheepishly confessed, "I'm sorry, Doc. She's my friend and neighbor. And of course you're right, her dog is as healthy as can be. But Dr. Vest thought it would be a masterful trick to play on you."

Showing off with one of his evil cackles, Rich said he couldn't stand the idea that I'd have a free afternoon with the boys. "When Rachel told me what you were doing, I couldn't resist."

I had to admit it was one of his more devilish pranks. But Natty was the one who froze up, continuing to blush. He wasn't yet accustomed to participating in the extraordinary lengths Rich would go in an attempt to pull off a practical joke. So I decided to initiate him by taking their trick one step further. Pretending to be angry, I said, "Dr. Horton, this was a serious breach of trust, so I'm afraid I have no choice but to consider firing you."

Natty didn't know if I was serious or not, so he turned to Rich. "Am I really going to be fired?"

"On a cold day in hell," Rich said, knowing I was bluffing.

"Are you sure?" asked Natty

Playing this out to the end, I turned without another word, grabbed my hat and walked toward my truck. I needed to get back to the store.

Pulling up to Karen's shop, I saw that the front door was wide open. I hadn't been gone that long, but the boys had taken over. Red was running the cash register while Laurel waited on customers. Danny was vacuuming the colonel's ashes off the carpet, and Cyrus was dusting shelves. Not one of these guys was qualified to be running a retail business— but they were actually having the time of their lives.

I was almost afraid to ask what had happened while I was gone.

"Hi, Doc," yelled Cyrus as he folded up the card table. "This store stuff is kinda fun. We sold a saddle, two pair of boots, and a hoof pick."

"And...and? Tell me...how did you do with the colonel? Did y'all treat him like the Good Book says?" I was anxious to know.

Quickly glancing around, I saw that the ugly saddle pad with the silver fringe was nowhere in sight. Punching the buttons on the register to open it, Red pulled out a check and waved it in front of me. It was for $1,000. I couldn't believe that my longtime professional friends had turned into such con artists.

"Yep, we remembered the words of the Good Book," said Danny, "We saw a stranger...and took him in."

We were sure the colonel would always think he'd gotten a great deal on the best saddle pad in the state.

After we sprayed air freshener throughout the store, my buddies went on home feeling mighty smug and content. And I went back to Meadow Creek to feed and water our clinic animals.

The power was back on that evening just as Karen came home from her show. And I waited for the questions, but got none. All she asked was, "Did you hear about the twisters in west Texas today?"

I felt like saying, "No, but you should have seen the four tornadoes in your store."

For some reason, she never mentioned the card game or even the sizable boost to her cash flow. Since she never brought it up, I didn't volunteer anything. It's possible she knew we were up to 'no good', and she didn't want to know about it. She wouldn't have approved.

It would be another two years before the four medics and I would have time again to goof off—and maybe even resume our aborted attempt to play a few simple hands of poker.

The Garlic Twins

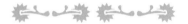

A faint scent permeated the air, and I figured either Rich or Natty had just ordered a garlic pizza for our ten-minute lunch break. Instead, Hanna-Belle Huntley called out from the front desk. Waving a card over her head, she breathlessly announced, "Hey, Doc...I gotcha another postcard from them gals in Europe."

Hanna-Belle had been our postal carrier for over twenty years, and was like a part of the family—especially since we knew she read everything that wasn't sealed with super-glue. I had the feeling that if I ever moved, she would personally track me down to hand-deliver whatever notes, letters or packages came from the two ladies she'd come to know only through their brief and unusual scribbling.

Quickly glancing at the postmark, I teased her, saying, "Let's see...this looks like a tall oil derrick in the middle of some big city."

Overly excited, Hanna-Belle blurted, "No, Doc...that's the famous Eiffel Tower in Paris, France."

For years now—every month—at least one or two postcards arrived from Bernice and Ethel Martucci. Even special letters and greeting cards came on birthdays and holidays. And every item that arrived had the odor of garlic lingering on it. The women wrote from just about every country they were living in at the time: Greece, Italy, Spain, and Germany. Of course, the cards weren't intended to be from Bernice and Ethel. They signed off each note with, 'From Tarzan and Jane'—their two Mexican Chihuahuas— along with the dogs' personalized, inked paw prints.

Bernice, Ethel's mother, was probably approaching ninety. And from photos they'd send, it was clear to see that she still wore her hair in a favorite poofy style. Though plainly clad, as was typical of many Italian women of her age, she nonetheless enjoyed coloring her cheeks a bright pink. It wasn't as noticeable until she got older. Then her round face took on the look of a painted doll's mask. One other constant adornment that never changed was the chain of fresh garlic bulbs worn around her neck. Supposedly, it helped relieve her arthritis pain. I'm not sure it worked, but she believed in garlic as a cure for just about everything.

Bernice was only fifteen when her only daughter Ethel was born. She gave birth while on the ship that brought her and her new husband from the Port of Naples to Ellis Island in New York.

Domineering and outspoken, Bernice always had a somewhat dismissive attitude toward her daughter. In her mother's shadow, Ethel grew up to be a shy and quiet woman. She was close to her dad, though, and even looked like him. They shared the same fair complexion and light hair; a vivid contrast to her mother's dark, classic Mediterranean looks. Unfortunately, her father Luca passed away at forty-five. I never knew—and didn't want to ask—what had happened to him. As a hard working and practical man, he was a great believer in putting a hefty portion of his salary toward life insurance. After his demise, mother and daughter were able to live and travel comfortably. And I often thought it was fortunate that Ethel never had to work, since she found it so difficult to carry on a conversation with people she didn't know well. I'd like to think that this was behind her father's motive to set aside such a nest egg.

As I held their latest card, permeated with the distinct scent, I reminisced to Hanna-Belle about the first time I'd met the Martucci family. "Luca was a first-rate electrician and did all the necessary electrical work to prepare us for the opening of our Twin Oaks medical facility. The fellow had an easy-going temperament and was fun to have around. He spoke English fluently, and must have learned it well before leaving Italy. It was during the first week of my practice that Luca introduced me to Bernice and Ethel, who brought in their twelve-year-old Chihuahua for an examination. The old dog's name was 'It'. Unfortunately, I had to tell them that their pet had a serious heart murmur."

Hanna-Belle shifted her mail pouch off her shoulder
to set it on the counter. It looked like she was about to settle
in for the afternoon as she took off her sunglasses. Cleaning
a lens on the shirttail edge of her gray-blue uniform, she
listened patiently.

"Their little dog suffered from congestive heart failure,
and I could treat him for that. But my challenges with the
Martucci family were more complex. Ethel was able to speak
some broken English, but her mother only spoke Italian…in
an unintelligible dialect that sounded like gibberish to me. I
had to marvel at the odd, but charming duo. Neither woman
could understand me, but both would be anxious to tell me
about 'It' and his symptoms of ill health. Luca didn't stay to
translate, since he was always on a job deadline. I also think
he felt this was the 'women's work'.

"I wish you could have seen it, Hanna. Using
pantomime as best she could, Bernice talked fast, as if I
could understand her. And using her fingers to gesture, she
described the dog's chronic cough by pointing to her own
throat, then making a hacking sound. Ethel would then
translate her mother's hand motions for me by repeating
everything in her broken English. She'd look into my face
to see if I understood her. I'd get the gist of what they
were saying, but only understood *daaga* for dog, and *seecka*
for sick."

Hanna-Belle shook her head, giggling. For some
reason, she wanted to know everything there was to know
about these Martucci women.

The strongest memory of that first meeting, of course, was the overwhelming smell of garlic, because even 'It' had two bulbs hanging on his collar. When I pointed to the bulbs, and to my nose, Ethel said, "Walking off *fleeesees*." At the time, it was fairly common for dog owners to know that garlic, in some form, helped control flea infestations.

"As sweet as these two eccentric ladies were, they came close to driving me crazy for the next four years. They'd call me on the phone every single day with a health report: "...eats *goodie*" or "coughs *leetle*" or "poops fine."

Hanna-Belle slapped her knee like she always did when she laughed, "They called every day?"

"Every morning at exactly eight o'clock," I said. "In fact, at a dinner gathering once, I was telling an attorney friend about them, and jokingly asked him if he had any ideas on how to avoid this ritual of theirs." He simply said, "Send them a bill for consultation."

"I felt uncomfortable doing that, but I tried it anyway, sending them a brief, friendly note along with a bill. The following week, they sent me ten dollars for the consulting fees. At the same time, the attorney sent me his bill for fifty bucks. There's a lesson in here somewhere, but I'm still not sure what it is.

"I continued to treat 'It', keeping the aging pooch on regular cardiac medication. He remained a constant source of delight to the women, until he eventually died peacefully in his sleep at the age of seventeen.

Bernice and Ethel were completely lost without their baby. So a few months after his passing, they went to the local animal-rescue center and adopted two Mexican Chihuahuas from the same litter. Naming them 'Tarzan' and 'Jane', Bernice and Ethel lovingly nursed the emaciated pups through a bellyful of worms and a spell of diarrhea. After that, the 'Linguini Duo', as I'd sometimes call them, spoiled the tiny dogs in ways that were hard to understand."

Hanna-Belle's timing on her route was always thrown off on days when she'd stay to visit with us. And I sometimes wondered what excuse she gave to her central station when she was late coming in at the end of the day. She seemed in no hurry to leave, so I finished telling her about Tarzan and Jane.

"Bernice and Ethel were both good seamstresses. And they made small lace sheets and satin-covered pillows for a baby's crib that Tarzan and Jane slept in. The dogs even sat in highchairs at the dining table in order to share meals with their 'famiglia'. Since they were the Italian duo's constant companions, Bernice even arranged to have special baby car seats made for them. The gals also made tiny necklaces of garlic for them, despite the fact that I was now giving the Chihuahuas medicinal tablets which no longer made the garlic necessary.

"I liked Jane especially. She was a lovable little pooch. But Tarzan was different, and seemed to have a split personality. When his owners were present, he was as gentle as could be. But whenever he needed to be boarded here at the clinic, he'd turn into a Devil Dog. After being nipped one too many times, I didn't dare run the risk of putting my hand in his cage. He could even bite through our lead-lined X-ray gloves. It was strange. Even if no one came near him, he'd lock his teeth on to the cage bars and snarl. Jane, on the other hand, rarely barked. She'd cuddle for hours, while making contented humming sounds almost like a cat's purr.

"Tracy thought she understood Tarzan, and said he was stubbornly rebelling at being put into a cage environment instead of his fancy digs at home. Since the animals' comfort was always Tracy's goal, whenever they came in she'd try to see what arrangement would work best for them. She ended up making an exception for these little tan dogs: They had their own separate quarters in an extra large cage so they could be together. Among other things, their home-away-from-home had soft carpeting...along with the satin pillows from their own crib. I had to admit that all of this seemed to substantially ease Tarzan's jangled nerves.

"We got to be pretty close with these two dogs, since they'd stay with us whenever Bernice and Ethel traveled for short periods of time. But the ladies were in a dither when they decided to close their house down and live in Italy indefinitely—using that country as a base to continue traveling. They couldn't bear to leave their two cherubs behind. So I suggested they take the pups with them. I'd prepare the necessary travel papers, and Tracy would do the research on which countries would either not allow animals, or would need to have them quarantined—something Bernice and Ethel would never stand for."

"So," Tracy added, "...we've been getting letters ever since, but we'll probably never see them again...though I still miss Jane, and even Tarzan. He was just too smart. And, even with special care, he never liked having to put up with us rather than being pampered by the ladies. I'd be the same way, too."

Finally turning to leave, Hanna-Belle was brimming with questions. "Can you figure why every postcard still smells? I'm curious as to why they're still using so much of the stuff after all these years. Them dogs don't need it anymore. And how come Bernice's Italian doctor doesn't give her somethin' else for her arthritis? Old habits die hard, I'm guessin'."

Throughout the years, I always thought Hanna-Belle's personal service was above and beyond the call of duty. But now I realized that she looked forward to the garlic-smelling cards. The notes were brief, of course, but the photos were outstanding and told more about the places than the two women ever could. Some were even the jumbo-sized cards. Hanna-Belle loved seeing those pictures of foreign places she'd probably never see. In a way, Bernice and Ethel had become her adopted 'pen pals'. And after having the cards on our bulletin board for a while, we'd give them to her. We believe she was keeping a scrapbook, though she'd never admit it.

The regular arrival of notes from the Garlic Twins eventually slowed down, then stopped. We assumed Bernice passed away. She was undoubtedly the instigator for most of the communications. And, knowing Ethel, we'd like to believe that she's still traveling with Tarzan and Jane, and letting them order 'Room Service' rather than writing to us.

We often wonder whatever happened to the four of them. So we keep one postcard, the one from Paris, on our wall as a reminder. In a mix of broken English and Italian—like all their notes—it reads:

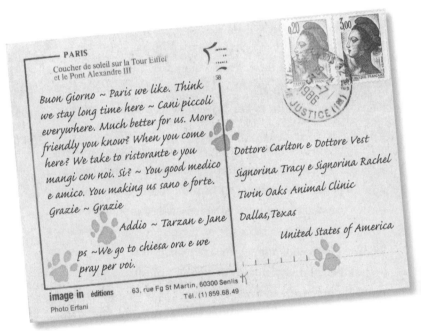

PARIS
Coucher de soleil sur la Tour Eiffel
et le Pont Alexandre III

Buon Giorno ~ Paris we like. Think we stay long time here ~ Cani piccoli everywhere. Much better for us. More friendly you know? When you come here? We take to ristorante e you mangi con noi. Si? ~ You good medico e amico. You making us sano e forte. Grazie ~ Grazie

Addio ~ Tarzan e Jane

ps ~We go to chiesa ora e we pray per voi.

Dottore Carlton e Dottore Vest
Signorina Tracy e Signorina Rachel
Twin Oaks Animal Clinic
Dallas, Texas
United States of America

image in éditions   63, rue Fg St Martin, 60300 Senlis
Tél. (1) 859.68.49
Photo Erfani

6

Who Knew?

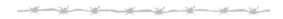

"Thank god, one of our boarders didn't show up," Dr. Vest said with relief. "There ain't no more room in the inn."

It was that time of year again, Christmas.

But it didn't matter if it was Memorial Day, Thanksgiving or Presidents Day. Even with two clinics open, all our boarding cages were filled. It seemed as though every canine and feline in Dallas came to stay with us. Their owners were "off for the holidays." And whether they went to a resort in Santa Fe, skiing in Idaho, or home to family in Utah…it meant we had their beloved pets for at least four to five days.

Through the years, everyone on our staff knew better than to plan anything special until after the last critter had gone home. And our families knew celebrations would wait. It was a call for 'all-hands-on-deck'. Every mother, son or cousin pitched in to perform his or her assignments. The kids would take scheduled turns in walking and exercising the dogs. And moms and daughters would give personal attention to the cats…finicky felines who never took well to being in a cage under any condition. The holiday symphony of barking and meowing sounds that echoed throughout our corridors came to mean Christmas to us—even more than hearing 'Jingle Bells' or 'White Christmas' playing on the radio.

When my partner asked K.C. what he'd gotten for Christmas, my son said, "Don't know, yet. We don't open our presents 'til the dogs are walked and the kitties are fed. Dad says that Santa doesn't come to our house unless we're all here at the clinic."

"Take these leashes, K.C.," I said, "…and walk those three next…that large poodle, the Beagle pup, and Jasper over there, the old grey Scottie with white whiskers. Your mom will be walking behind you with the three blond cocker spaniels."

When Rachel answered the phone, I knew it had to be an emergency. Those are the only calls we get on the holidays. "Joyce Pinkerton's two cats are comin' in," she announced.

It took Joyce only five minutes to show up with the family's two eight-month-old kittens, Mita and Rojo. And their problem could have been predicted. Every year, on cue, kittens encounter the same dangers. Mita, formally 'Micontesita', had chewed through an electrical cord for the tree lights, and Rojo had sliced the cleavage of his upper lip on an ornament.

Mita was hissing and growling, so Tracy carefully wrapped her front claws in a towel. The roof of the kitten's mouth had been cut and burned by the hot circuit wires. I couldn't tell just how badly she was hurt until I'd given her a sedative to sleep.

Rojo, or 'Don Gato El Rojo', as Joyce preferred to have him listed, stayed with Rachel and waited his turn with restlessness. I'll never know why so many people feel obliged to give their pets such fancy monikers.

As she explained what happened, Joyce said something we've probably heard a thousand times. But that fact never diminished the reality of the consequences. "Doc, when I brought our Christmas tree into the living room, both cats went wild. The hair on their backs went straight up and they hissed at it. Then after just ten minutes of wonder and exploring, they spent hours tumbling and playing in the lower branches. These are city cats, Doc, they've never seen a tree, much less climbed one."

Continuing to describe their plight, Joyce said, "During one of their romps, the lights flicked off. Mita's whiskers were singed, and Rojo still had part of a bulb in his mouth, but there was blood on his chin."

With Mita now asleep, I asked Tracy for a suture pack and began the stitching in Mita's clefted palate. "Joyce, cosmetically, I can repair this vertical burn...but she'll need to spend the night to sleep off the sedative. And there shouldn't be a scar. But give her soft foods for a few days...even baby food should do well."

Tracy scooped up the sleeping bundle of grey fur and took Mita into our hospital section. I asked her to tell Rachel to bring Rojo in next.

"Oh, Doc, Rojo's such a love!" Joyce chimed in.

Rachel was grimacing as she came in holding the beautiful Maine Coon cat, his long haircoat of grey and white swirls still bristling. "Mrs. Pinkerton, your 'love' just bit me."

When Dr. Vest came by to see if we needed any help, he studied the tiny puncture on Rachel's thumb, and dismissed it, "That's just his way of sayin' Merry Christmas." Knowing enough to don a pair of thick leather gloves, my partner held the cat still, while Tracy washed the dried blood from Rojo's lip and smeared topical antibiotic on the small cut.

As Joyce kept apologizing for Rojo's behavior, I reassured her, "He's okay now, so you can take him home. But we'll see you again tomorrow when you pick up Mita."

She was still feeling guilty when she came in the following day to get Mita. "Thank you all so much. But I'm so sorry Rojo bit you, Rachel, it's really not like him."

Coming back from his afternoon dog-walking trip, K.C. seemed tuckered out, "Dad, how much longer are we gonna be here? Santa's waitin' on us."

★ ★ ★ ★ ★

A few days later, as we were readying more dogs and cats for their departure, Rachel began complaining about not feeling well. She even asked to go home early, something this spunky gal had never asked before. At first, we thought she was exhausted from the holiday workload. But when she said she felt like she had the flu, we took her temperature. She did indeed have a fever of 102 degrees, along with chills and muscle aches.

Rachel had already been to her doctor, but he confirmed that it wasn't the flu. So I asked her if she'd let me call her personal physician to discuss the case. I'd known Dr. Scott Holcomb for years. In fact, he would occasionally sit in on our rare poker parties.

"Her symptoms mimic everything but influenza," Dr. Holcomb said. "So we checked her for Lyme disease, rheumatoid arthritis, and even malaria. Her EKG and blood chemistry profiles were normal. All we could find was an unidentified bacillus on the blood culture. With all the animals you deal with there, this may be…"

"It could be Cat Scratch Fever…that unidentified bacillus is probably the bacterial cause," I added.

"You think that's possible?" asked Scott, " I've heard of the condition, but I've never seen it."

"I've had the disease myself," I responded. "So has Dr. Vest. And judging from our experience, Rachel's symptoms will probably subside in a few days on tetracycline. But thirty days of antibiotics are usually needed to kill the bacillus. In all the years of my practice, I've never known a vet who wasn't aware of the disease."

"Since this illness is not that uncommon, I'll be showing the blood culture to my colleagues, and making sure the full information is dispersed throughout our medical system. But, Doc, we'll need to get some extensive research done on this. In other words, perhaps a vaccine would need to be developed. Do you think you're immune now?" Scott asked.

"I just don't know. It's one of those things that somehow never gets talked about or written about. I suppose there are some people who would overreact and get rid of their cats…and that would be a sad situation."

This holiday proved to be quite different after all. Rachel recovered quickly, but would be telling her friends about this episode for some time to come. Scott's e-mails and newsletters would get the medical community up to speed on a not-so-rare illness—one that's probably been around for centuries.

And our boisterous dog and cat choir finally left for home, with promises to return again on the next three-day holiday…when everyone else is either out of school or off from work. Everyone, that is, except us.

7

A.J. Strikes Again

I missed it all. While I'd been away presenting an invitational lecture to veterinary students in College Station, Dr. Vest had another run-in with our old nemesis, A.J. Hall. Rachel tried to give me bits and pieces of the unbelievable story over the phone. So I was more than anxious to get all the sordid details from my partner as soon as I returned.

Extreme heat, poor pasture grasses, and bad advice from local horse traders resulted in a lot of summer calls from owners reporting sick horses with upset stomachs. And they feared the worst—that it might be colic. What little I'd heard on this case was that a gelding was in severe pain, and somehow A.J. was involved. All I could think of was that every single encounter with A.J. turned into a nightmare.

Colic isn't just a bellyache. It's a disease with literally dozens of causes and symptoms. The painful episodes can come from serious gastrointestinal bloat and reduced blood circulation to the stomach. Other causes can include a twisted bowel, coiled intestines and obstruction by foreign bodies…as well as grain overload, parasitic damage, gastritis, colitis, hemorrhage, trauma and cancer. And that's the short list.

Dr. Vest is a man of the utmost compassion and understanding when it comes to our patients' needs. So it was a surprise to find him so angry that he could hardly speak. He tried to fill me in: "Phyllis Grimes called on one of those days when you were gone, and our case load was heavy and hectic. I was already behind schedule, but she sounded disturbed when she told me that her horse might be ill."

"Doc Vest, Banjo is obviously uncomfortable. His eyes are dull, and he's not eating or drinking. He's just moping around with his nose on the ground like he's lost his best friend. Doctor, sometimes he'll even roll on his back, then quickly stand and paw the ground."

Sighing heavily, Rich said, "Then Phyllis had two more comments that made smoke come out of my ears. She said, 'Doc, A.J. looked at Banjo earlier and thought he might be getting the colic."

My heart sank, and I had a bad premonition. But I wanted to lighten my partner's mood, so I lamely joked. "Getting the colic is like getting a *little* pregnant. Are you sure she said *the* A.J. Hall? The one with the grey stubbly beard and potbelly, who always wears a ratty straw hat and a dirty green shirt? That A.J. Hall?"

Rich groaned, "Yep…you know that's him, that son-of-a-so-'n-so horse trader who will forever be a thorn in our side."

Since I also knew Phyllis quite well, I wondered how she had hooked up with A.J. We'd see her often at the clinic when she came in to get shots for her bouncy Yorkshire terrier, Alf, and Pepsi, her grumpy white Persian. Since she kept Banjo out at the River Bend Stables, I'd go out there regularly. And with the help of her stable manager, I'd worm and vaccinate her fourteen-year-old Appaloosa gelding. Banjo was an alert, handsome red roan with a spotted rump. It was a shame she didn't ride him more. A charming housewife and mother of two from the North Dallas suburbs, she tried to be a 'super mom'. Striving to be as perfect as possible in everything she did, she was fond of telling her friends and family about her superb horsemanship. In truth, she seldom rode and knew very little about equine husbandry, though she did make sure Banjo was always well cared for. And that's all that mattered to me.

"Don't tell me A.J. gave Banjo any medicines, did he?" I'm not sure I even wanted to hear the answer.

Hesitating, Rich began explaining just the first part of a hair-raising ordeal. "No, at ten o'clock this morning, he told her that Banjo wasn't that bad. But he advised her to rub turpentine on his navel, then jump him over several creeks."

This was a perfect case of the 'blind leading the blind', and I imagined a scenario of Phyllis trying to leap over puddles of water, while Banjo refused to move. I could even hear her saying, "Doc, there ain't no creeks out here."

Smiling to myself, I continued to listen as Dr. Vest repeated Phyllis' explanation. "Doc, I've been dragging him around on the end of a lead rope. He's sweating and wobbling...and I'm exhausted. But he's no better. What else can I do? A.J.'s on his way back out here. I called him first, since we used to keep Banjo at his stables. But what do I tell him?"

"I tried," said Rich, "to muster some professionalism before I answered her question. But what came out was, 'Phyllis, you tell A.J. to leave Banjo alone, and not lay a finger on him. Tell him he's an ol' quack, and that I'm on my way.' But she suddenly cried out that Banjo was going down, and she screamed, 'Hurry, Doc!'"

"I told her to try to keep him standing, no matter what."

It was probably true that A.J. had seen his share of horses with colic. Unfortunately, though well-meaning, his backwoods' mentality and strange ideas often led to disaster.

Apparently, Banjo was on the ground in pain when A.J. headed out to the rescue. But Dr. Vest was in hot pursuit... in a frantic rush to beat A.J. before the ol' side-buster could get there to inflict some treatment that could be potentially dangerous.

Rich described what happened next. "Phyllis was in tears when I arrived. And a small crowd had gathered at the corner of the yellow barn. But I couldn't see Banjo anywhere. All I heard was a loud, crusty voice commanding, 'Turn the water on.' Phyllis saw me and yelled, 'He's dying!' As I rushed forward, the crowd parted. In the center of the circle laid Banjo. He was lying on his side with his head tightly snubbed to the base of a large round post. And A.J. was kneeling by the horse's rigid tail. 'Hold 'im down, boys, and turn the water on!' A.J. ordered."

As Rich said this, my blood went cold. This was even worse than anything I'd expected.

"Four men, two on Banjo's neck and two on his body, pinned the horse's torso down as A.J. feverishly worked and Banjo struggled.

"Mud flew, hooves pawed, and people gawked in disbelief. I could see Banjo's four white stockings flailing aimlessly. 'The water's on!' someone yelled. I was aghast!"

"My gawd, what did you do?" I choked out.

"I raced into the mayhem. Banjo was exhibiting most of the clinical signs of colic. He was sweating and grinding his teeth. But his left eye was swollen shut from banging his head against that damn post. 'What are y'all doin?' I yelled. 'Who did this?' I shouted again at the top of my lungs.

"A.J. stood up and smugly replied, 'I did,' pretending to take offense that I could even question his expertise, 'Why, what's it to ya?'

"Because you're gonna kill that poor beast, you son-of-a..." Rich's voice cracked as he tried to continue. He still had difficulty controlling his emotions when thinking about A.J.'s ineptness.

Rich slowly attempted to finish the story, "I couldn't believe my eyes, Doc. Water gushed onto the ground. A water hose—of all things—extended from the poor gelding's rectum to the faucet. I immediately grabbed the rubber hose and began extracting it. Eight feet or more of the hose slipped from Banjo's lower bowel. And the force of the water sprayed like a fire hose when the nozzle hit the dirt. I jumped to cut Banjo's head loose from the post. Yet, A.J. stood there defending his logic, saying, 'He was dehydrated, Doc. His guts were blocked.'"

I was breathless at this point, "Then what happened?"

"Banjo tried to stand, but fell. He cut his right eyebrow, and blood coated the side of his face. Phyllis began screaming as watery feces squirted from the horse's colon. Then Banjo stood, but fell again. He landed like a ton-of-bricks. I grabbed his halter, administered two injections, and passed the stomach tube. Large amounts of fermented fluids and gases billowed out onto the ground. Then Banjo calmed, as I kept murmuring to him, 'Good job, boy, good job.'"

"The crowed applauded in amazement when Banjo stood again, though he was somewhat wobbly," Rich said. "But ol' A.J. continued to defend his treatment by loudly announcing, 'I guess my fire-hydrant enema worked…it's a good thing I unlocked his bowels for ya, Doc.'"

My partner's jaw was set and his hand was clenched in a fist as he shook his head. "Then, of all things, Phyllis acted like she approved of what A.J. did, by saying, 'Oh, thank you, A.J., thank you.' She kept repeating it 'til all the folks standing around started clapping again."

Forcing a sad smile, Rich went on, "Doc, the horse was not impacted or dehydrated. Banjo was bloated because he'd broken into the stable's feed bin and had a feast for himself. But my explanation fell on deaf ears. A.J. made himself out to be a hero. I don't understand…when something happens, why do people call everyone else in town before they call a vet who has actual medical knowledge and experience?"

I didn't have an answer. For the past twenty years, not a day has gone by that I haven't asked myself the same question.

It was unusual to see Dr. Vest dejected like this. Patting him on the back, I consoled him as best I could, "Try not to worry about this, Rich. I've been snookered by A.J. in the same way…and more than once! I know it feels lousy, but he ain't gonna change. At least you got there in time, and did what you had to do. Another sixty seconds of that 'water treatment' would have been fatal. But Banjo's fine now. And that's all that counts."

As I drifted off to sleep that night, I thought again about Rich's day…and how often I, too, came home totally exhausted and dispirited. I realized then, with great clarity, that it was rarely the work on animals that took its toll. It was coping with a few of the owners that could plumb wear you down. I vowed, then, that in my next talk to vet students, I'd warn them about any unusual owner behavior they might encounter. Maybe I'd even add some sort of joke…telling them that, along with their medical degree, they'll need a second degree in psychiatry.

8

Where's the Time?

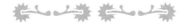

We were locked into a modern-day 24/7 dilemma. With both clinics running at full speed, finding any time to spend with Karen became close to impossible. Between her long hours at the tack shop and my time on the road for farm calls, our only communication was through brief phone chats. And literally half of the time away was a result of emergency calls. That old quote applies to anyone in business: "Poor planning on a client's part ends up constituting an emergency on your part." But when it comes to medical care, these emergencies can't be put off until the next day.

So, with some surprise, we found ourselves in the same place at the same time on a rare Sunday afternoon. We decided to cruise the back roads, with just meandering in mind—and no schedules to keep. Since it was a special day, we wore dressy outfits rather than our usual smocks and jeans.

Karen's leather skirt made her look like a vaquero drover, and my fancy pinstriped shirt looked like it belonged to a celebrity-dude. But, it was fun—and our only real outing in months.

It was a perfect autumn day. Heading out across the Grapevine Dam, we pulled over to the side of the road to take in the vista of tall stands of oaks and maples. Breezes whipped through falling golden leaves, sending them spiraling down to the warm earth.

We turned onto a heavily used jeep trail that would take us to the lake's edge. Some folks lazed about on the decks of drifting sailboats, while couples on the beach-strand baked in the sun. A few kids were trying to water ski, while their father stood nearby building a fire for a family barbeque. To our tired eyes, this was as close to an idyllic sight as possible.

My pager went off...abruptly ending the daydream before it had a chance to begin. When a second page came in, I cringed, knowing this day would be no different than any other. I must have sounded pathetic when I told Karen I'd take her back to the house, and make my return call. She just grinned, saying, "Well, it was great while it lasted. But think I'll tag along on your appointment...since I'd rather see you working than not see you at all."

My mobile hadn't been functioning since the day before when a rambunctious colt tried to chew off the antenna. So I needed to stop at the first phone we could find. Spotting a small shack with a faded 'Joe's Bait Shop' sign hanging out front, we figured this might be the place. Telling

Karen I'd be just a minute, I jumped out of Ol' Blue's cab
and headed toward the store. A tin bell jangled over my head
as I tugged away on the handle of the creaky screen door.
It opened only about halfway before stalling and scraping
another scratch in the already deeply worn grooves of the
wood-plank porch. I had to duck as I walked into the shop to
keep from getting entangled in a web of paraphernalia. Lures,
trout lines, stuffed bass mounts, and minnow nets hung down
from the rafters to the very top of the cluttered and dusty
display cases.

In a strange way, I felt at home. Something about
the place reminded me of my old college dorm room. And I
don't know why because my roommate and I were never this
messy. Lingering tobacco smoke from a stale roll of Kentucky
leaves filled the room. And, in the corner, a cedar chair with
frayed wickerwork was still rocking with no one in it. Looking
around for signs of life, I spotted one of those antique wall
phones with a megaphone mouthpiece. The hand crank
needed for operation was still attached. It had to be working.

Emerging from the side of a ceiling-high, red Coke
machine, an unshaven, elderly gent held his arms out in
greeting, "What can I getcha, sonny?"

Joe's sudden appearance caught me by surprise, and I
stood there speechless, completely forgetting why I was there.
Hunched over and squinting below the bifocal line of his
glasses, he stood there quietly looking me up and down. He
knew I was no fisherman, and I'm sure he was curious about
my fancy duds. He was obviously the proprietor of the store.

But with his crumpled and stained Hells Angels sweatshirt
stretched tightly around his belly, I found it hard to tell
whether he was 75 or 105.

"Joe?" I asked. "Joe, I just need change for the phone."

Spitting his stubby cigar to the floor, he kneeled
behind what might have been a trinket counter, and pulled
out a Mexican-tiled coin box. "Might hav'it...might not,"
he said, smiling an almost toothless grin, since only three or
four of his front teeth were evident. After his smoker's cough
brought on a brief choking spell, he huskily obliged, "If ya ask
me nice, I might have two quarters and one Indianhead nickel
...for a dollar."

Reaching in my pocket, I pulled out a crisp new
bill and placed it on the counter. Joe opened his palm with
the coins, and shakily counted out fifty-two cents. Not
mentioning the missing nickel, I asked, "Fish been bitin'?"

"Nibblin' fair," he mumbled as he shuffled to his
rickety rocker and resumed whittling. By the look of the
mini-mountain of shavings on the floor, he might well have
been sitting in that one spot for fifty years.

As I dropped my quarter into the phone slot, Joe
amiably offered instructions. "Might need to bang that
receiver on the post there. It ain't been workin' like it use'ta.
Nope...none too good. And don't be surprised if they cain't
hear ya. Kinda like the fishin'. Sometimes they bite and
sometimes they don't."

Sure enough, when Luther Milsap answered, his voice
sounded like it was coming from the bottom of a well. Yelling

into the cone-shaped speaker, I shouted, "Luther, is that you?" Then I strained to hear the faint sounds at the other end.

When Joe told me to hammer the receiver on the lid of the minnow bucket, I did, and Luther's voice was suddenly clear. The foreman of the Longbranch Dude Ranch was able to explain his emergency, "Doc, Water Lou's done cut his leg."

"Is it bleeding?" I hollered as though Luther was in the next county.

"No...but ya don't hav'ta yell. Doc, where are you?"

"I'm leaning over a tank of minnows," I laughed. "I'll explain later...but you can expect us there in about ten minutes."

As I fumbled with Joe's last quarter, it slipped out of my grasp into the algae filled tank. Grumbling to myself, "Dang, this is ridiculous," I rolled up my sleeve and quickly plunged my arm into the stagnant water...while wondering how all those small fish could even survive in it. Sifting through the silt, I was able to retrieve not only my quarter, but two others, as well. There's no telling how much money may have been buried under the sand.

Calling out from the shop's door, since she couldn't open it, Karen asked what was taking so long. When I waved for her to go back, she knew not to say more. On my way out of the shop, the crooked door got stuck in its track again, but Joe kept on whittling...cheerfully bantering, "Y'all come back now, ya hear?"

I turned Ol' Blue onto the blacktop road and made speed toward the corrals at Luther's and Mark's dude ranch for tourists.

Passing under the Longbranch's arched gateway made of wagon wheels, we circled around to the chuck wagon where the two would be working. Luther and his partner, Mark, or 'Tex' as the visitors liked to call him, had just finished baking up enough biscuits for a crowd. Uncommonly tall at six-foot-six, Luther was an impressive sight as he stood there stirring beans in an enormous cast iron pot. Tex was preparing thick gravy in a ceramic skillet. And both boys were so skinny that we had to assume they never ate their own greasy chow.

The partners were expecting their usual group of weekend travelers who were coming out to experience the real *Wild West*. And Luther and Tex were already in their costumed-gear, with the ever-present red and white kerchiefs tied around their necks.

"We'll be right with ya, Doc," bellowed Tex, when he saw our truck pull up.

Wheeling Ol' Blue past the water trough, I saw a glimpse of Water Lou and stopped. His ribs were showing and he was more potbellied than when I was last here. His ears were pinned back, and he was showing great discomfort. This seasoned rent-line horse was probably not much younger than his two aging owners. Now lame, Water Lou tried to pivot at my approach, but had to hobble instead.

"What happened here?" I asked the boys as they came up the path.

In a slow drawl, Tex said, "He cut it last Tuesday."

"No, it was Wednesday," corrected Luther.

Pointing to a rusty plow blade in the middle of the paddock, Tex again said, "He cut it on that...Tuesday night."

Quick to anger, Luther snatched his hat off and threw it to the ground, "No...dernit, Tex, he cut it on the edge of the barn, right over yonder...on Wednesday mornin'."

Karen never could take their constant bickering. A horsewoman through and through, her priorities were always on target. "It doesn't matter where or when, let's just take care of the horse!"

I began to walk toward Water Lou, while the boys continued to argue and point in different directions. But I was overwhelmed by a foul stench that kept getting stronger and stronger. At first, I thought it was coming from the boys' manure-soaked boots, but then identified the familiar odor of decaying tissue.

Gently patting Water Lou and muttering to him, I looked down to see the gaping wound. Across the bulb of his heel was an open gash that had maggots churning in and out of the laceration. Karen turned her eyes away, and I kept shaking my head in disbelief.

Still holding the wooden spoon he was cooking with, Tex shooed stable flies away from the raw cut, splattering gravy in every direction. I almost gagged thinking about his unsuspecting dinner guests. After sticking the spoon down the yoke of his boot with its handle jutting out, he became defensive about the gelding's condition, "Damn flies...Doc,

I sprinkled bakin' soda on the cut Monday, but these flies just..."

"No...dernit," Luther interrupted, "...that was last Friday."

I figured the gelding's cut was a week old, but, at this point, it wouldn't do any good to say anything. Karen and I whispered to one another, wondering why it took so many days for them to see the horse's problem.

"Can ya fix 'im, Doc?" asked Luther

"Cain't spend no damn money on 'im, though," Tex added.

Swearing to myself, I told them I needed a bucket right away.

"I'll get the blue one."

"No, Tex...the red one's better."

"But that one's in the barn."

"No...it's in the shed!" Luther said, after losing his temper again.

Joining one another in a search, they kept up their non-stop quarreling. Rummaging through the clutter, Tex exclaimed, "I'll be damned, here's them pair of hoof nippers we lost." And, of course, Luther contradicted him by saying he knew where they were all the time.

Tapping me on the shoulder, Karen motioned toward a green bucket next to the water trough.

"Here's one, boys," Karen said, picking it up and turning it over to examine it. Then, winking at me, she pointed to the bottom.

"Yep, that's just the one I was looking for," Tex announced.

"Me, too," Luther had to say.

"But, guys," I said, "There's a hole in the bottom of that one."

"Then it'll havta be the red one."

"No..."

We needed to put an end to this absurd fiasco. The jousting duo reminded me of Abbot and Costello, and their old comedy routines.

Still, I found it hard to believe that Luther and Tex were grown men with a business. "Stop, enough already..." I said. "Luther, you hold on to Water Lou's lead rope."

"I'll hold 'im," said Tex.

"But he asked me."

"You're an ass."

"Am not."

"Are, too."

As the boys circled poor ol' Water Lou, kicking up dust and continuing to fret, the horse's jaw locked. And Water Lou's eyes widened into a glare as the squabbling men took turns jerking away his lead rope. Balancing on three legs, Water Lou was in too much pain to put up with his owners' antics anymore.

Karen and I had both seen that look in a horse before. Following me to the truck, my wife quietly said, "Horses don't forget. That gelding is going to get even with those two...and very soon."

I grabbled my stainless steel bucket and filled it with a soothing medicated solution to cleanse Water Lou's wound —but not before loading a syringe with a tranquilizer.

At the sight of my full bucket, the boys asked, "Whatcha gonna do, Doc?"

"I'm going to let Water Lou soak for awhile."

"I'll do it, Doc...give me the bucket," Tex insisted.

Suddenly water and medicine splashed through the air, as both men fought over the bucket, spilling out healing solution. The two were crouched around the gelding's hindquarters, when Karen pulled on my sleeve, "This is it... we best step aside."

While my plan was to coax the horse into letting his sore heel soak in the relieving lotion, it was apparent Tex and Luther had a different approach. When I stepped a few paces back, Luther seized a tight grip on the gelding's cannon and ankle, while Tex slam-dunked the bucket of liquid over the sensitive flesh. Water Lou's ears flattened, his rump dropped... and in one smooth move, he bolted, kicked and whirled, sending my pail sailing through the air. "Look out!" one of the boys yelled.

Tex limped away, groaning, "He got me in the thigh!"

"Here," Luther ordered, "...come back and do the leg and I'll hold the bucket this time. They exchanged places and asked me for more medicine. It was the first time they had agreed on anything since we got there. After mixing another batch of medicinal lotion, and handing them the bucket, I moved back to an even greater distance.

They went through the same grasping and dunking routine, and it looked like Water Lou wouldn't resist. "We got 'im this time," they proclaimed. The horse allowed his hoof to be guided to the ground, then waited for them to let go of the bucket. He stood quiet and, for a moment, I thought their method might work. But I should have known better.

Luther was standing behind the horse feeling smug. Then he began bragging, "I guess we showed 'im alright."

Karen and I knew what was coming. We only had to wait a few minutes. Water Lou's head dropped. We waited another minute. Maggot larvae began floating out of his wound to the top of the bucket's solution. After five minutes, I was surprised when Tex and Luther shook hands, saying "We done it!" Water Lou wasn't moving a muscle. Then, the horse took aim. His tail twitched and his nostrils flared. In a flash, his hooves went flying. WHAM. In an instant, Water Lou had made his move work with precision. Both boys were down. Tex was lying flat on his back, out cold. And, Luther, doubled up in pain with my bucket embedded in his groin, was on his side moaning, "Ouch...ouch...eeow!" Water Lou turned his head toward them neighing and nickering, seemingly satisfied. At that moment, I'd have given anything if more folks could have witnessed Water Lou's calculated maneuver. It would have helped put an end to any lingering myth that horses were not smart.

Patting the gelding's neck, I crooned "Whoa, good boy." Water Lou had been neglected and overworked for so many years that I was amazed by his undiminished spirit. His ears perked as he let me inject his vein and wrap his wound. "This cut needs a light cast," I told the boys, as Tex wobbled to his knees and Luther slowly stood up.

Still dazed, the dueling pair avoided my eyes, and spoke directly to Karen, "Ma'am, can you send us a bill... please?" They knew that I knew they were faking.

When we finally drove out through the wagon-wheel gate, I kept asking Karen the same question, "What could I say?"

"You'll never get paid. Those boys just barely get by with their seasonal tourist business...and they've come to expect free vet work from you."

I went on changing Water Lou's bandage every week until his wound healed completely. I actually extended his care longer than needed, just to give him a deserved rest before he was put out to work again...carting one tourist after another up and down the same rocky trails, dozens of times a day. This was indeed an expense the two cowpokes could ill afford. But I considered offering to have our clinic take the horse off their hands in exchange for all medical bills they had accumulated over the years. After all, we now had our Equine Senior facility where Water Lou could retire.

"I know you feel the animals come first," Karen would chide, "...but you can't go on working for nothing."

"I also have another plan," I said. "The boys, and maybe a couple of our other strapped clients, can work off their debt by taking care of your shop one day a week, preferably Sunday. They'd have the chance to pay their bills, and we'd have a chance to spend more Sundays together. As K.C. would say, 'It's a win-win situation'. What can you say to that?"

"With any of your other clients, I'd say that's a good possibility. But with that combative, not-so-funny comedy team of 'Luther and Tex'...never, never...never!"

So it was settled...partially. Since one of our clients had just lost her job in a company downsizing, she was anxious for a chance to pay off the cost of her German shepherd's hip surgery. She liked the idea of working at the shop every other Sunday for the short period of time needed. And though this wouldn't promise a lot of future free time for Karen and me —at least it was a beginning.

9

Preacher-man

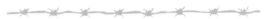

My truck pitched and bucked up and down over the terraces of Bobby Erwin's fifty-acre field. Fighting the steering wheel, I tried to keep a straight path as I aimed Ol' Blue through a newly constructed wood gate and down over the sloping land. Doing his best to navigate me, Bobby was standing at the Trinity River bottom and waving his arms over his head —looking every bit like a signalman on the flight deck of an aircraft carrier.

The hefty fellow jumped around frenetically, trying to keep my attention. I didn't see the patient he had phoned us about, and assumed the lactating cow must be on the ground somewhere, hidden by the tall winter wheat. A dozen of his heifers and a few steers were grazing in the lush green pasture behind him.

I reminded myself to be on my best behavior, since Bobby was not only a part-time rancher, but also a fulltime preacher. I came rumbling to a stop at the bottom of the hill, when he called out, "Doc, Lulu is over here...but her calf, Boo, is way off yonder playing." At that moment, I wondered if all his cows had names, but figured I'd asked him later.

I'd only met Reverend Erwin once, while attending a baseball game at my son's high school. But Karen and K.C. talked about him often and seemed to think highly of him. My wife considered him artistic. She said that during Halloween festivities, he'd carve so many unusual jack-o'-lanterns that folks kidded him about being the 'Pumpkin Picasso'.

The chaplain appeared pale with worry over Lulu. From the sight of his sweat-drenched overalls, he must have been trying to help her in any way possible. Though he had attempted to prop Lulu up on her chest with two bales of hay underneath her, she continued to lie flat on her side, unable to move. Her head and neck were extended and her forelegs were drawn. As her breathing became labored, the preacher panicked. Grasping his forehead, he then began to nervously run his fingers through the few strands of hair he had left on his head. "Oh, my God, please don't let her die," he said softly.

Kneeling down next to Lulu and Reverend Bob, I could tell that the cow was in bad shape. Lulu couldn't control the spasms of her facial muscles and legs. Though she had little strength, I saw where the involuntary thrashing of her hooves had torn through the earth. No wonder the preacher was beside himself. Lulu tried to raise her fluttering eyelids to see me, but her eyeballs also twitched uncontrollably. I proceeded with a quick examination: Her rectal temperature was normal. She didn't have a bloated abdomen. Her tongue was pink, though hanging from the side of her mouth. And she had no indication of excessive salivation or teeth grinding.

I considered tetanus or rabies, but neither condition fit my gut feeling. So I started to ask Bob if his cattle were on any mineral blocks. Just then, Lulu's eyes rolled back, and she began to convulse wildly.

"Oh, Lord...no!" moaned the reverend, as he stopped to pray silently. A first time mother, Lulu bellowed out for her bull calf. Echoing his mother's call, Boo came bounding up from the creek. Crashing through the weeds in a frenzy, he got to her side and kept squalling, *Baaa...baaa.*

With his hands clenched into fists, Bob blurted, "Damn it, Doc, what is it...what's wrong with her? Damn!... I mean darn...sorry, Doc, sorry." Briefly taken aback by the pastor's unexpected outburst, I told him what I thought had stricken Lulu.

"Reverend Bob, I believe Lulu has a case of grass tetany—an extremely severe calcium imbalance. It's really fortunate you found her when you did." I raced to my truck to fetch the right medicines, and kept racking my brain trying to remember the specific clinical symptoms of the ailment. Grass tetany leads to low magnesium and hypoglycemia. The rich cereal grasses have such a sky-high level of potassium and nitrogen that other essential absorptions are blocked.

The subsequent deficiency in vital minerals and nutrients can then lead to an acute nervous disorder. Looking out over the scattered herd, I knew it was only a matter of time before the other cows would be affected, too.

As I rushed back to Lulu with a bottle of Mag-Cal solution, plus a four-inch I.V. catheter and a rubber intravenous tube...I gave a silent thanks to the heavens that I had the correct medications. Pressing my knee behind Lulu's ear to secure her head, I threaded the 12-gauge stylet into the opening of her jugular and began chugging the electrolytes into her vascular system.

I held the inverted bottle as high as I could, and Lulu's explosive convulsions diminished. Greatly relieved, I turned to Bob, "We were lucky this time, Reverend...but it's not unusual to find cows of this breed succumbing to tetany without warning." Even Lulu's minor episodes subsided as the life-saving fluids balanced out her deficiencies.

With her strength returning, Lulu tried to get up on her legs. "Whoa, girl, whoa, you're not ready to stand yet. But I'll letcha roll over onto your chest." As I said that, Boo began nudging his mother. And her instinct to care for her calf took over. With sudden alertness, she struggled to her feet even though I tried to keep her quiet a while longer. But I was no match for her 1200 pounds of determination. Her calf began nursing contentedly, and the sight was enough to reassure Pastor Bob that all was well again.

Still a bit guilty, Bobby said, "I hope you can forgive my outburst, Doc. But I was in the army for several years before I took up the Lord's work. And I guess...well...even so, I should be able to control my language by now. But I... well." He stuttered, trying to explain himself. And I thought it was unusual, and even refreshing, to hear a clergyman be tongue-tied. Up until now, the ones I knew were all preachy, non-stop talkers.

I had to interrupt, "You needn't explain anything to me...I understand." Bobby blushed and lowered his head. I admired the man, but knew he was being too hard on himself. "Besides," I added, "...maybe God didn't hear you."

Feeling fully vigorous once again, Lulu bellowed loudly and trotted off with Boo trailing behind her. "Bobby... I mean Reverend Erwin...the next important step is to protect the rest of your herd. You need to dry-lot the cattle with bales of prairie grass for a few days. Then, add magnesium supplements to their grain, or given 'em mineral blocks to lick on. And try not to worry so much. I don't think God bothers to pay much mind to us ranchers, preachers...or vets."

Now laughing, and obviously grateful, Bobby continued shaking my hand 'til I thought it would come off. "Thank ya, Doc. But at least God was watching out for Lulu. As the bible says, 'the meek shall inherit the earth'."

I never knew what that meant, and I'm not sure Bobby knew either. Maybe it meant Lulu and Boo would outlive all of us. And that's okay with me.

Heading out the farm road, I continued to watch Bobby in my rearview mirror as he gathered his small herd, moving them toward their clean metal-paneled pens. Looking every bit like a true shepherd, he was happily calling out to each cow, "Gertrude...shoo, shoo. Bubba Son, git-up there. C'mon, Bill, move it. And Angel Face...let's go!"

I turned onto to the asphalt highway, and waved to the preacher-man as I headed back to town. I now had the answer to one of my questions. He did, indeed, give a personal name to each of his cows. What I still didn't know is how he could tell them apart. These were Charolais cows from France, and they had distinctive characteristics. They were very large, and very white...all white.

Musing on the pastor and his 'pets', I thought about joining Karen and K.C. next Sunday at the Baptist minister's service. I wanted to hear a little of what this goodhearted fellow had to say from the pulpit. Then, after church, maybe I'd get him to tell me how he's able to know the difference between each of his beautiful...and identical bovines.

10

Reunion

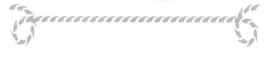

It was already dusk when I approached Dallas. It had been a cool and windy day—a welcome change after weeks of sweltering heat out on the farms during the recent cattle plague that had rocked the state. My associates, Rich and Natty, stayed behind to continue working. But after making a promise to my boy that I'd make the opening night of his school play, there was no way I could miss it. He'd gone through weeks of rehearsals in preparing for a lead part in Shakespeare's *King Lear*. And I hadn't been around enough to hear a single one of his lines.

As I quickly pulled up to the front of the clinic, Ol' Blue's screeching tires must have signaled my approach. I could see Karen pacing up and down in the lobby, looking at her watch. And, in his colorful knight's costume, my son just stood there blankly staring out of the window. He must have been overwhelmed with stage fright. Thinking I could ease his opening night jitters, I dashed in and made a sweeping bow with a theatrical flourish of my hat. "At your command, my lord, I hastened my arrival for this auspicious eve."

Getting into the spirit, K.C. began, "Where hath thou been, good sir?" Before he could go on, we were startled by an odd tapping sound. Everyone turned around to see what it was. The faint, repetitive tapping continued and seemed to be coming from one of the paneled windowpanes next to our entranceway. The front door was open, and a few clients were still at the reception desk. So it would have been apparent to anyone outside that the clinic was open. Out of curiosity, my son went to investigate. And we heard him saying to someone, "Can we help you, mister?"

In a hesitant, low voice, the person said, "Doc, *izzdat* you, Doc?"

I knew the voice...and quickly went to greet the elderly gent standing there. But he backed away from the entrance, as though he didn't wish to intrude. Over his crumpled clothes was a faded Mexican serape. But as he clenched and unclenched a frayed, almost shapeless, baseball cap in his hands, there was no question as to who he was. Though now stooped over with age, 'Johnny' was a legend in our parts —and my boyhood hero. I was happy to see him, but, at the same time, my heart went out to him. His wispy scrub of white hair was combed close to his black head, and I figured he must be at least 95 by now. No one ever knew his real age. And, in fact, no one knew him by any other name but Johnny...or 'Negro Johnny' as he was known in the 1940s.

Grabbing his frail arm and shaking his hand vigorously, I invited him inside, "Well...I declare, Johnny...it's really you! Come in, come in. K.C., I want you to meet a very special gentleman."

My son took Johnny's trembling hand, just as Karen joined in to give the old man a hug...also urging him to come inside.

"Yes sir...yes ma'am...but don't mean to be no bother."

Though we hadn't had a chance to speak to Johnny in years, there were times when we'd see him ambling through the streets of town with his wagon and two mules. From time to time, he'd pick up odd jobs from folks who had businesses on Market Lane. From what I heard, he always did fine work. And, as was his nature, he generally put in more time than he had to.

Johnny peeked inside with some apprehension, and I assumed he'd never been in a veterinary hospital before. Still, he carefully wiped his shoes on the doormat and came in.

As he raised his head to look at me, I was startled to see that his eyes were clouded over by cataracts. Concerned as to why he hadn't had medical attention, I started to talk to him about it. But he had other things on his mind. "It's *mah* mule...he ain't good, Doc. He's bitin' his side." Then dropping his eyes again, he mumbled repeatedly, "*Ah* com'da fetch ya. Jesse ain't good...not good at all."

Appearing to be short of breath, Johnny paused a moment, and I realized how difficult this trip must have been for him. He would have had to walk the full six miles from his cabin to our clinic.

In an effort to let me know how urgent the visit was, he raised his hands in emphasis, his fingers noticeably buckled with arthritis. But he was trying to speak out clearly, "He ain't good, Doc...ailin' bad, I'ma sure of it!"

The man was so weak that Karen was afraid he might drop over. "Johnny, please sit down and rest for a moment."

Steadying himself by grabbing the back of our bench, his shoulders swayed a little, but he was firm, "Ain't got time... *mah* mule be sickly."

"Please, Johnny...just for a minute," I added emphatically.

The old man slowly moved to the doorway again to retrieve the two prized possessions that he was never seen without: an old wooden baseball slugger, stained and notched with wear, and an ageless four-finger fielder's mitt...stuffed with cotton. With the glove dangling from its wide end, he laid the bat across his shoulder. That was his trademark. And just as he took that stance, he stood upright, looking like the Johnny I remembered—proud, athletic—and ready to play ball. Then he suddenly wilted again...and sat heavily on the bench.

Momentarily forgetting about Shakespeare, my son's eyes were fixed on the cracked leathers of Johnny's mitt. Since the old man was resting for a bit, it seemed like the right time to tell K.C. more about my connection with Johnny.

"I was just a kid about nine years old. And growing up in these southern plains was a whole lot different than it is now. Every Monday night, a bunch of us would either walk or ride our bikes across miles of dirt roads to the cattle arena at the Samuel Ranch."

Karen added, "That place was just up the road from where we are now."

"Anyway, we'd watch the cowboys rope and brand the ranch's steers. It was all the entertainment we had then in this small town of fifteen hundred souls."

"It was fifteen thousand souls," Karen laughed, as she corrected my tendency toward melodramatic stories.

"Anyway, there were no video games—only radio listening and fence watching. We'd sit on that arena fence for hours and hours.

"Our own Pete Channel, already a roping whiz, would see us there so often, sitting astride the top wood rail, that he decided to do something for us. In his usual no-nonsense way, he began our boy's baseball team—long before anyone called it 'Little League'. He made all the arrangements with Mr. Samuel. So when the roping arena wasn't being used, it became our diamond. The bases were made of any makeshift things we could find; even a couple of dried cow pies were used once.

"There were just enough boys for two teams...and that's all we needed. We really didn't know much about the game, but it didn't keep us from playing our hearts out. Pete couldn't be with us all the time, since he was already becoming popular on the rodeo circuit. So he did something better. He found us the best possible coach—Johnny. With his expertise and exuberance for the game, Johnny guided us through daily practice in everything from fielding to pitching."

Looking up at the clock, K.C. reminded me of the time, "We gotta leave in twenty minutes, Dad…if I'm going to make the curtain."

But I continued, "You know how nice the folks in this town are, don't you? Well, back then, many of them were not so nice, even intolerant. Behind our backs, they'd frown and whisper to one another such things as, 'What's a black man going to teach them boys?' But we didn't care, and Johnny didn't care. He never let us down.

"Johnny had a phenomenal instinct for the game. And Pete told us that the rumors about him were true. He was not only a terrific shortstop, but also a world-class batter. He'd have played in the major leagues, too, if it hadn't been for the color of his skin. A few years after Johnny retired from the Negro League, that unjust barrier was finally broken by the legendary Jackie Robinson when he joined the Brooklyn Dodgers in 1947."

My son stopped me, "No way…there couldn't have been both black teams *and* white teams."

"Yep, there were. Not only that…but even after the majors had integrated, there were still ten southern states that wouldn't let their white leagues play against the black teams. There's even a book about the whole story called *Let Them Play*. You can get it at the library." Then, noticing

Johnny dozing off on the bench, we walked to the other side of the room to keep from disturbing him.

"Even as he got older, anywhere kids would be cracking a bat...he'd show up. It was awe-inspiring to see Johnny hit every single pitch out of the arena. He was just that good. When a game was over, he'd hitch his mules to a flatbed, steel-wheeled cart for his trip home.

Every now and then, we'd invite him to our house to visit and have dinner. But, instead, he would only stop by the back door. Each time, he was asked to come inside, and each time, he'd shyly refuse. So my mother would fix him a plate of food to take home. Other folks did the same. He'd been paid so little for all his years of coaching, that families felt this was the least they could do to repay him for introducing all of us to the sport of baseball. Shoot, son, everybody came to love that old man."

As I said that, I patted Johnny's shoulder. His white stubble-bearded chin rested on his chest, and his palms lay open on his lap as he snoozed. Since it was day's end, Rachel and Tracy stopped to listen before leaving for home. And my ever-present rottweiler, Aggie, exhausted from her work in the country, curled up on the bench next to Johnny with her head on his knee.

"Unfortunately, Johnny never had any schooling, so he can't read or write...and he can't count money. Whenever he goes into Noble's Donut Shop down on the square, he'll buy a pastry by holding out a handful of change to Julia, the waitress, telling her to take what she needs. Most times, she takes less than he owes. He'll graciously nod and say, 'Thank ya, ma'am...*ah* hopes ya took a lil' extra for yer trouble'.

"I don't know of anyone who took advantage of him. Folks knew he never asked for anything for himself. And they wanted to do things for him. You know Jed Silver, our local contractor, don't you? Well, Jed and I were in the boys' league at the same time. A few years back, Jed wanted to build Johnny a more comfortable home with indoor plumbing. But Johnny was too proud and independent to accept help."

My son took a long look at Johnny...and then at the clock. "Dad...why don't Mom and I leave for my play now. But you should stay and go help Johnny's mule...'cause it's more important. Okay?"

In his regal costume, K.C. looked twice his thirteen years. But, when it came to wisdom, he was older than anyone I knew.

I gave my boy a hug and wished him luck with another stage-like bow, as Karen whisked him out the door.

No Finer Man

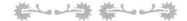

ently shaking the old gentleman, I whispered, "Johnny? Johnny...let's go see your mule now."

Mumbling as he awakened, he kept repeating, "Jesse's sickly."

Grabbing Johnny's bat and glove, I helped the old pro to his feet before leading him out our side door to my truck. He shakily pointed his finger down the road. "Yes, sir," I said, "I know where you live, Johnny." I didn't think he could remember me from the many dozens of boys he taught to swing a bat or field a grounder. And that didn't matter... because I remembered him.

Johnny balked when I opened the truck door. I'm not sure he'd ever been in a truck. Holding on to his upper arm, I helped him up into the cab. Quietly, he announced, "*Ah* don't trust these *thangs...ah* prefer to be walkin'. *Ah* walks fine, ya know. Better than most."

"I know you do...I know. But we'll get to your mule much faster this way."

While patting his thighs, he tried to make a point, "*Mah* legs be fine...strong." Then, as Ol' Blue's engine fired up noisily, Johnny abruptly stopped talking. Gripping the edges of the seat, he didn't say another word until we reached his one-room log cabin ten minutes later.

In the dark, my headlights illuminated Johnny's favorite place—under a willow tree next to his small shelter. He kept the same old hand-woven cane chair he'd been partial to for years. And even when the seat shredded through, he took care of filling the holes with foam rubber—just like he took care of everything for himself. He loved sitting in that chair under the tree's shade, and leaning back against the wall of the dwelling he built. This was his home.

I'd been here as a boy, and it all came back to me. It was obvious that Johnny appreciated this heavily treed, tranquil area. He was diligent about keeping a tiny, but bountiful, vegetable garden of corn, tomatoes, squash and beans. His dozen or so chickens roamed free, and as we drove in I could hear them rustling down by the whimsical outhouse...also constructed by Johnny. Curiously balanced between two aging oaks with gnarled limbs, I was amazed that it never toppled over.

I don't know if Johnny owned these few acres. It's possible that Pete gave the parcel to him as part payment for his coaching services. No one bothered him out in the country. There wasn't much here, other than a few remaining track-beds holding up a half-dozen rusting boxcars once belonging to the now defunct Rock Island Railroad. Up the hill behind his place was an abandoned cemetery with its tilted and broken tombstones almost obliterated by weeds and high grasses.

On our arrival, I could smell tortillas and beans. And I was glad to know Johnny was still cooking his own meals. I realized, though, that bringing a vet out to see his mule was probably the only medical help he'd ever asked for. I also wondered what he and the animals did during severe weather. With no pens or sheds for the critters, I could only assume Johnny brought them all into the cabin with him. That would, of course, be something he'd do.

Deciding to leave most of Ol' Blue's lights on to see my way around, I helped Johnny get down from the truck. One mule, the 'molly', nickered a welcome as we made our way over to the trees where they were tethered. She looked just fine. But the 'john' was pawing the ground in pain. It didn't take long to see that Jesse had colic. He stood there drenched in sweat. And his gums were a muddy grey. Being tortured by his abdominal cramps, Jesse was near death.

Holding his coal-oil lantern close to me, Johnny watched closely as I rectally palpated the mule. The lantern's flickering wick provided insufficient light, and even my truck lights weren't enough to help me see properly. So I moved Ol' Blue closer to the trees and snapped on the powerful high-bright search beams. For once, I was glad these were installed.

After confirming the massive impaction on the left side of Jesse's abdomen, I cringed and told Johnny, "Jesse's bowels are blocked."

But he seemed hard of hearing, so I shouted, "His gut's are blocked."

The sweet man got straight to the point, "Can ya unblock 'em?"

I yelled again, "I'll try!" And Johnny nodded. I didn't hold out much hope, but I had to try my damndest. Sally and Jessie were everything to Johnny. I stood there as he held their necks, whispering to them. Then he spoke gently into Jesse's ear, "Doc here's come ta help ya...not hurtcha, *mah* li'l Jesse."

I tried breaking down the bowel's obstruction by manual compression...but it didn't work. Then, using the nasogastric tube, I pumped a gallon of mineral oil and stool softeners into Jesse's stomach. Resorting to stronger options, I also administered pain relievers and anti-spasmodic medications.

Though Johnny fretted through all of this, he became entranced by the procedures. I threaded a six-inch intravenous catheter into Jesse's neck vein. One liter of fluids ran into his jugular vein...then another. As the fluids continued to drip, Jesse stumbled, still in pain. "Where's all tha water goin'? Why are ya stickin' yer arm up his rear? Why's that *thang* in his neck? Is he gonna git better?" Trying to give Johnny straight answers to all his questions, I saw his eyes beginning to water when I used the stomach pump to drain fermented gasses from the mule's upper bowel. The smell was overpowering.

Knowing I needed a little time to see if anything would work, I felt some distraction would help us both. "Johnny, why don't you take Sally down to the creek to slake off her thirst...okay?"

I should have known the old man was aware enough to know why I suggested this. After Sally was untied, she trotted down to the shallow stream that ran alongside the tracks. And Johnny slowly followed her. In the distance, I could see the orange glimmer from his lantern. Then he turned right to take a walk, and Sally tagged after him.

Two hours passed while I kept fighting to keep Jesse on his feet. He'd respond briefly to pain relievers, then collapse. I kept monitoring the solid mass in his small colon as I gave him more drugs. With each palpation, though, it seemed my efforts were futile. The only fluctuation in Jesse's symptoms was from good, to bad, to worse.

My hopes were gone. I'd run out of tricks. Bottles, stomach tubes, exam sleeves, needles and syringes littered the hood of my truck, and gastric secretions soaked the ground. With blood up to my elbows from running supportive fluid drips, I was totally frustrated. Then, Jesse went down...again.

In complete exhaustion, I sat on the ground beside the mule. There was nothing else I could do. Johnny had returned and knew not to say anything more. Though Jesse's eyes stared down the hill, it was an empty stare. His ears were flopped— not only signs of sedation, but also dejection. As the mule lay there on his side, I knew he was dying. "Damn...I've failed!"

Without a word, Johnny started off toward the graveyard with Sally at his heels. I assumed he wanted to be alone with his thoughts. After five minutes, I heard a sharp sound. CRACK. In my weary state, I thought it sounded familiar. Then again, CRACK rang through the air. And Sally whinnied, *EE AW...EE AW.* I couldn't figure out what was happening until the retorts came sharply, one after the other, CRACK–CRACK.

I looked down at Jesse. His long ears perked up, and his eyes began to focus. The mule was still lying on his side. But he raised his head, and his front legs curled up under his chest. After a momentary silence, his muzzle dropped back to the ground.

CRACK–CRACK. Johnny was hitting 'home run' rocks with his trusty bat. In his infinite wisdom, he was doing for Jesse what my modern medical techniques couldn't do. The mule's head began to rise up slightly. I hollered, "Johnny, keep swinging!"

The old man heard me, and he began hitting rock after rock into the air with nonstop precision. Jesse's head rose again...and he tried to answer...*ee aw...ee aw.* CRACK–CRACK–CRACK. With every swing, Johnny smashed another piece of granite all the way to Oklahoma. The body of the prone mule in front of me tensed with excitement. I was elated. Jesse rolled up onto his chest and answered *EE AW...EE AW.* Jesse now fixed his eyes and ears on his master's silhouette at the top of the hill. "Swing!" I hollered, screaming the same words to Johnny that he once said to me when, as a kid, I stood frozen in the batter's box. "Keep swinging!"

The all-time greatest hitter heard my every word. He waved his glove high in the air to acknowledge me, and smacked another couple of rocks. CRACK–CRACK. Stretching his legs in front of his torso, Jesse sat. With the next CRACK, he drew his rear hooves together and began rocking back and forth, back and forth...trying to gather strength. Jumping to my feet, I grabbed his halter, "Come on, boy, come on. You can do it." He rocked four or five times, then stood... whinnying loudly, *EE AW*. Jesse's legs wobbled, but he was standing—on his own. Stretching into a sawhorse position, he began to stagger a bit—then straightened and walked forward. I couldn't believe my eyes.

The mule actually began strutting toward Johnny and Sally as they made their way down the hill. The slugger's pockets were bulging with rocks. And with every other step, he'd pitch one in the air and hit it with the distinctive crack. As the sound got louder and closer to us, Jesse got stronger. His muscles relaxed, and his tail was raised as high as his ears.

Johnny was feeling playful now, and hollered to his mule, "That's a'nuther home run for ya, Jesse!" He stopped to celebrate by smacking two more stones into the sky. Jesse answered, *EE AW...EE AW,* and began trotting. Then he stopped abruptly, and in a total physical release, finally sprayed out so much diarrhea that it sounded like a waterfall splashing against the flat boulders. We all felt such overwhelming relief from the noise that Jesse and Sally threw back their heads to whinny, and Johnny waved his arms back and forth, laughing.

I had to be sure the mule had actually beaten this illness. Patting him on the rump, I gathered his lead rope. Listening to his heart with my stethoscope, I was pleased to hear a normal rhythm. His eyes were now bright, and he even reached down to graze on a few sprigs of grass. As the pain relievers wore off, Jesse's gums turned pink again. For one last time, I felt the pelvic flexor. The obstruction was gone. "Thank God," I whispered to myself.

Johnny was so grateful that he stopped for a moment at the willow tree to say something private. Then he came over to me holding out a handful of change. Smiling with his usual wonderful grin, he said, "*Ah* owes ya, Doc. Take somethin' for tha' hard work 'n trouble we caused ya." Both mules were now shoving and nudging me in the back with their noses as I closed Johnny's hand.

"Weren't no trouble at all, Johnny. Besides...baseball did the curing."

"Take whatcha need, Doc," Johnny insisted, opening his hand again.

I needed to remember that this was a proud man, and I didn't want to insult him. So I started to take three nickels... then dropped them back into his open palm. "Wait, Johnny... I'll make you a deal. I'll always take care for your mules if you'll buy me a cup of coffee every Friday morning at Noble's Donuts."

The old slugger grew quiet. He was probably trying to figure out if this proposition was a good deal or not. Then he wagged his finger in a scolding manner, "Okay, Doc...*Ah'll* be there...but coffee ain't good for baseball players." I had to agree with him...and we shook hands on our deal.

Johnny kept his word. Every Friday at ten o'clock, we'd sit in the front window-booth of the donut shop. I'd have a hot chocolate, and Johnny would drink apple juice. As we both nibbled on the freshest buttermilk donuts ever made, we had ourselves some good long talks. Johnny was never late... not for five weeks. Then on the sixth, he didn't show up.

Mr. Samuel called me at the clinic that afternoon to say that he and Pete found my hero sitting in his cane chair, with his chin down on his chest as though he'd been sleeping. His bat and glove were still resting on his shoulder. And Jesse and Sally stood close to him, quiet and motionless.

There wasn't a person in our parts who didn't attend the funeral. In the eulogy, Mr. Samuel announced his donation of a piece of land to the town—that original arena where Johnny taught the game of baseball to so many kids. It would be called Johnny Porter's Little League Park. A sculpted piece of granite with an engraved plaque was positioned behind home plate to honor and commemorate our unforgettable coach. The inscription begins *'There was no finer man...'*

As promised to Johnny, I continue to look out for Sally and Jesse. And Pete lets me keep them on his grazing land behind the ball park. The mules seem to love the sounds coming from the field. It's always full of activity, with team games and kids running the bases. And whenever the crack of a bat is heard, Johnny's mules match the sound with their own inimitable baying and whinnying. They've become the players' two loudest fans.

Bleachers have replaced the ol' fence where we sat as boys. But, now, in the very same place, I find myself cheering on K.C. whenever he's up at bat. I know he can hear me hollering at the top of my lungs, "Keep swinging, son...keep swinging!" And I think of Johnny every time...

12

Canine Hypnotist

Brushing her dark hair away from her face, Jody Red Deer frowned with worry. "Hondo hasn't gotten any better. At first, I thought it was just a sprain, but he won't put his foot down anymore. And if I touch it, he cries out in pain." The lovely woman with soft Indian features then cradled Hondo's muzzle in her hands and looked into his eyes.

Trying to balance on three legs, the Australian Border collie hobbled into the exam room holding his right leg up away from the floor. And Jody explained, "Dr. Horton, Hondo disappeared for two days. And I felt something was seriously wrong, because he never misses his job. In fact he loves it so much that he's absolutely tireless. He finally came home last night, but as you can see...he's limping badly."

Dr. Horton knelt down and greeted the normally agile sheepdog by lightly scratching the fluffy grey and black hair on Hondo's broad chest. At the gentle touch, Hondo sniffed Natty's hand and gave him a big slurpy kiss on the cheek. His feathery tail thumped against the floor, and he blinked up at his newest acquaintance, showing one brown eye and one blue eye. Natty knew two different eye colors were common for the breed, and that these dogs had unusually sharp eyesight.

Dr. Horton hadn't had Border collies as patients before. But he'd heard so much about them that he was glad to finally get to know one—up close and personal. Running his hand down the back of the dog's ruggedly built body, Natty wrapped his arms under Hondo's flanks, and lifted the lean animal up and onto our Formica table. Having trouble gripping the slick surface, Hondo spread out his three good paws, flexed his right rear, and stood there like a tripod. While Natty closely studied the injured leg for any signs of lesions or trauma, he asked Jody if she thought he could have been hit by a car or kicked by another animal.

Jody said she was puzzled. "We're out in the country, so there are no roads or highways. And he's too fast and smart to ever be taken off guard by another animal. The mystery of all this is that Hondo is well known throughout the county as one of the best herders around. And he never stops...he'd work around the clock if he could. In fact, when his duties on the ranch are complete, he'll sometimes go over to the Davidson farm and herd their chickens. The owner, Jim, though he likes Hondo, is none too happy when his chickens get so nervous about being corralled into a corner that they don't lay the usual amount of eggs."

Dr. Horton continued his exam, and mentioned to Jody that he'd never seen a dog with such strong and hardy muscle tone. But he felt an abnormal grinding in Hondo's coxo-femoral joint when he tried to extend and rotate the hip socket. The working dog, usually tougher than leather on a boot, was reluctant to show pain. But Hondo yelped as Natty tried that specific manipulation.

"Jody, this breed may be prone to hip dysplasia, but that's not the case here...although Hondo does have a problem in his hip joint."

"How bad do you think it is? This guy is indispensable to us, and it's not in his nature to slow down for anything. If need be, he'd want to work on three legs. The greater the challenge, the better he likes it. That's just how strong his will is. And he can still boss the other animals because his main talent is in hypnotizing them."

Dr. Horton thought that Jody might be in denial about her dog's injury. "I don't understand...hypnotize? How's that possible?" Natty thought that this might be an Indian belief. Jody's American Indian heritage was impressive. She was the great granddaughter of Three Hawks—the famous Kiowa pathfinder whose exploits are vividly recounted in many history books. Jody and her father had inherited their ancestor's vast sheep ranch.

"You'll have to come out and watch him someday, Dr. Horton. Hondo can master any type of herd and any kind of animal. Many believe it's not only his physical prowess that helps him achieve dominance, but his ability to mesmerize animals with his eyes. As he crouches down before the animals and stares intensely—with laser-like focus—it's as though his mind and body become one with them. At that point, he has full command."

Dr. Horton may have been new in town, but the rest of us already knew of Hondo's reputation among farmers. And we heard that a few of them even paid Jody fees for the collie's hypnosis services, since he was able to accomplish a herding task in only a fraction of the time that it took other dogs.

Natty was entranced by this story and assured Jody he'd visit one day to see this for himself. But, as usual, he was direct, "First, I have to tell you that I don't know the extent of Hondo's injury. We'll need to get some X-rays. I expect that your canine ranch hand has had a blow of some kind...and he may have a fracture. If you can leave him here for an hour or so, we'll get him sedated and take the pictures. Then I'll give you a call with the results."

Jody quickly agreed, since she'd been on her lunch break and needed to rush back to work. A serious but amiable woman, she'd been employed by the Department of Interstate Commerce for several years as an accountant. We'd known her for some time, so Tracy couldn't resist kidding Jody as she was leaving. "How can you do so much and still stay on top of your ranch work? I'd say you're a workaholic...but, then, so is your dog."

Smiling a rare smile, Jody said, "You're right, I guess we're two of a kind."

Tracy held Hondo while Dr. Horton injected the necessary anesthetic that would relieve the dog's pain and allow for proper positioning on the radiology table. Two views of the hurt limb were taken from different angles in order to have a three-dimensional image of the pelvis. When Tracy slipped the resulting films against the viewing screen, Dr. Vest came in to peek at the results along with Natty.

Rich gulped hard when he saw the film, and pointed to the segmented lines of the shattered fracture. "Natty, you're a stellar surgeon, but this is going to need some difficult and sensitive work. I'm not sure I'd even take it on. I'd be inclined to bring in a specialist...though a hip replacement is out of the question with this broken socket."

"I know...but I can perform a head and neck ostectomy giving Hondo a chance to walk on all fours again. It's a long procedure, but I've done it before. And I need to call Jody right now and explain this to her."

"Whew! Your confidence never ceases to amaze me. But you know we'll be here to assist if you need us. I'll carry Hondo into surgery, while you talk to Jody. And, Tracy, come with me and we'll get the room ready for our young Dr. Horton."

Natty felt that Jody didn't understand what he was saying when he tried to repeat his discussion with Dr. Vest. So he explained it in another way, "Jody, we still don't know what caused this...it might have been a freak accident. We do know that on impact, the ball portion of the ball and socket hip joint shattered the pelvis bone before the head of the femur or ball dislocated and created breaks in the femoral neck which attaches the hip bone to the rest of the leg bone."

He thought he'd been perfectly clear, until Jody remarked, "What? Can you simplify that for me?"

"You probably remember part of the old song, 'Them Bones', that goes...*the ankle bone's connected to the leg bone —the leg bone's connected to the hip bone...*and so on." He even attempted to sing the phrases. Well, Jody, the leg bone ain't connecting to the hip bone anymore. Hondo needs major surgery, and..." Jody interrupted Natty before he went on further. She didn't need to hear anymore.

Always precise, the lady had exactly four questions for Dr. Horton: "Can you fix it? When will you begin the surgery? Can I make monthly payments to the clinic? And is it a simple surgery?"

"I can begin right away. No...it's not a simple operation. There are risks that there could be permanent nerve damage or a post-surgical infection." He didn't want Jody to have any doubts about the severity of this procedure.

After hesitating a moment, Jody softly said, "It doesn't sound like I'll be able to pick him up tomorrow."

Hondo was lying on his side under general anesthesia as the steady rhythms of the monitors tracked every beat of his heart. And Tracy began prepping him by clipping his sleek fur away from the area to be readied for the surgical incision.

"Jody, we'll need your consent to do what has to be done. You can either stop in to sign our form, or you can nod

twice on the phone and we'll consider *that* as your consent."
There was no sound on the other end for two breaths. After
Jody thanked Dr. Horton, he quietly added, "How 'bout I call
you back as soon as I'm done? And if it gets late, I'll call you
at home."

After donning his surgical gown, cap and mask, Natty
scrubbed and gloved his hands. Then after checking the
tracheal intubations and anesthesia maintenance, he began.
During the long complicated surgery that took two hours, Dr.
Horton displayed the finest surgical expertise possible. When
finished, he was pleased that he was able to avoid the major
sciatic nerve during closure and replacement of the muscular
attachments. The process would support formation of a false
joint as the pelvic fractures mended.

Already accustomed to two perfectionists like Dr. Vest
and me, Tracy was nonetheless visibly impressed. And unable
to contain herself, she impulsively planted a kiss on Natty's
cheek when they were done.

Natty felt certain that Hondo would be able to walk
and run again with his normal gait, though he'd be carrying
his leg up for a few weeks. Then, with gradual assurance, he'd
begin to bear full weight.

Anxious to let Jody know, he called her even before he
and Tracy took Hondo to his recovery cage. "Hondo will need
to take a little time for mending. And since he's not the kind
of guy that can stay still, we may consider giving him a mild
tranquilizer for a couple of days while he's here. After that, if
he has the company of someone who watches over him, he

should be his old self in four or five weeks. But I'll really need to see him once a week to be sure the healing is going well."

Jody's usual controlled responses came undone. She'd been fearful of the worst. And her relief was overwhelming as she stammered a bit trying to regain her composure and express her gratitude to our colleague. Then, pulling herself together, she said, "Dr. Horton, it seems the origin of this problem may no longer be so strange. Remember Jim, the farmer I told you about? He called me about twenty minutes ago to say he saw Hondo laid up in his barn yesterday, and didn't know how long he'd been there. But the dog was covered in mud. Since Jim was unable to reach me by phone, he cleaned Hondo up a bit, put him in his truck and brought him to my place knowing I'd see him as soon as I got home. Jim guessed that Hondo was trying to gather all of the farm's sixty pigs into one place...but in the process of rapidly moving around in the slippery mud of their waller, he probably twisted and slid...taking a nasty fall."

Natty couldn't keep from grinning as he tried to visualize the scene, "That sure makes sense, doesn't it? And it would account for the unusual fractures. By the way, Jody, when your boy's ready, all of us here are going to take you up on your invitation to go out to the ranch and watch your canine-Svengali do his stuff!"

Just then, Dr. Vest cracked opened the door and gave a whistle, congratulating Natty on the superb operation. "And when you're all done in here, come next door and see what I found. You're not going to believe it."

13

Treasure Hunt

Dancing a fast two-step down the hallway, my partner sang out to everyone within earshot, "Ladies and gents, we have ourselves a patient that's the most expensive feline known to man."

Though Natty was getting accustomed to Rich's antics, he remained on his guard to avoid becoming ensnared in one more practical joke. Just the same, out of curiosity, he wanted to see this rare breed. Envisioning an exotic Abyssinian or one of the Devon rex cats he'd read about, Natty told Rich he'd take a look.

Replying almost too gleefully, Rich said, "Sure...go on in and see this priceless cat...though he'll be slowly awakening from anesthesia. His owner, Nick Turner, is still in there with him."

Entering the exam room, Natty first saw Nick leaning against the surgery table, speaking in low tones to a strange lump of fur. But Dr. Horton thought he was in the wrong room. The kitten on the table was only about seven months old...and very odd looking. He was a steel-gray longhair with white whiskers. But he had a flat nose and big jowls. Initially, Natty thought he might be an alley cat, especially when Nick kept calling him 'Scrapper'. He wondered why anyone would give such a name to any of the unusual breeds.

The funny-looking cat began licking his lips, though his eyes were still closed and his body remained motionless. Rich didn't mention what surgery was done, so Natty quickly looked over the instruments that were used. A spay hook, thumb forceps, a hemostat, and gauze squares were spread out on the table, and both an endotracheal tube and esophageal feeding tube lay on the countertop. For the life of him, Natty couldn't understand why such a vast array of instruments was out. After closely examining Scrapper, he became even more puzzled since there were no signs that surgery had taken place: no wounds, no cuts, no stitching...no nothing.

Scrapper's eyelids flickered as he slowly began to wake, and Nick seemed joyful, "I can't tell you how glad I am to know that our guy's okay now. After all, this is a $6,000 animal."

The cat's tail had been shaved in such a way as to resemble the distinct look of a lion's tail: close-cropped until the bushy tuft at the very end. Natty could see that Scrapper was part Persian, but, oddly, most of his hair-coat was matted and scruffy as if he were an outdoor cat.

Having heard that Nick was the high school gym instructor, Natty presumed he must be a responsible fellow. So while rubbing Scrapper's chest waiting for the kitten to regain consciousness, Natty couldn't help but ask the coach why his pet had been sedated.

"Well, his tail was one big knotted fur ball, and my wife and I couldn't comb it...so we shaved it instead. I brought him here because he'd been gagging for three days."

"He was choking for three days before you brought him in?" asked an astonished Dr. Horton.

Adjusting the long whistle strap draped around his neck, Nick said, "I know that was too long to wait. I actually started to bring him in sooner, but he only gagged when he tried eating. He was playful during the rest of the time, so I thought that whatever was bothering him would pass."

Sleepy, but finally awake, Scrapper sat up on the table purring loudly and pushing his head against Nick's arm. Still confused, Dr. Horton asked Nick why both he and Dr. Vest were acting so giddy about this whole medical procedure... whatever it was. At that moment, Rich strolled in, still grinning.

"Alright, Rich, what's been going on in here? This kitty ain't no pure breed, there's been no surgery...and yet you've got every medical instrument known to man displayed." Folding his arms across his chest and forcing a smile, Natty leaned back against the counter, and waited for an explanation.

"As you can see, he looks fine," began Dr. Vest, "...and on my first exam, all his vital signs were normal. But when

I attempted to inspect the oral cavity, Scrapper strongly objected by diverting me with his front claws extended in attack mode. I tried a couple of times, but he fought me off so intensely that I figured he should be sedated if I was going to see the inside of his mouth. Even after he was asleep, I searched but couldn't see anything. I was looking for a possible pharyngeal ulcer or a bad tooth."

"Fine," said Natty, "...but that doesn't tell me why you're both so happy."

"I'll tell you, I'll tell you. I was about to consider radiographs to see if a foreign object was present. But first, I inserted the endotracheal tube to make sure the windpipe was clear. Then I passed the small feeding tube down Scrapper's esophagus to be certain there was no blockage to the stomach." Rich hesitated and Natty knew he was stalling. Rich always made use of a dramatic pause before delivering his punch line.

"Then...I saw two faint, strange lines running beside his larynx." With his usual flair, Rich opened Scrapper's mouth to illustrate. "They looked like strings of mucus...but something told me they weren't."

"Are you going to tell me what you found, or not?"

With obvious enjoyment, Rich continued, "Using the tissue forceps, I teased out what I thought was a piece of string. It was hard to identify due to the salivation in the back of the cat's pharynx. But, lo-and-behold, a loop of something shiny started to lift out from the side of Scrapper's tongue. I used the spay hook to grasp the loop, then fetched the hemostat and gauze to catch whatever I was about to bring out."

Now tapping his foot with impatience, Natty said, "I swear, Rich, your stories get longer and longer. Will you please get to the point?"

Dr. Vest said, "Well, I didn't rightly know what we had. There was a raw place under Scrapper's tongue, and two fine thread-like twines were leading deep down in his throat to a gnarled clump of something."

Nodding his head, Nick said, "It was green and awful looking."

Rich was getting to his finish line, "With a steady, gingerly tug, I was able to drag the glob out. Coiling it in the palm of my hand, I..."

Stopping to put his hand on Natty's shoulder, he went on, "I rushed over to the sink and washed it clean."

Coach Turner took it from there, "That thing sparkled with brilliance, even under the water. There, in Doc's hand, was my wife's diamond solitaire necklace—worth $6,000. It had been a wedding gift from her mom and dad."

Describing the circumstances, Nick said, "The fine chain had broken. So to be sure she wouldn't lose it before taking it in for repair, Sandra tied dental floss to the chain links and looped it through the tiny clasp on the diamond stud. I still don't know how the cat got hold of it. But he likes to jump up on my wife's dresser and bat around any baubles he sees. Sandra often finds earrings and lipsticks scattered all over the floor. You know how young cats are...they get a little wild when they play. But for him to actually swallow such a large gem is unbelievable. I can't wait to tell Sandra. She's been worried sick wondering how her diamond could have disappeared. You can imagine how relieved I am that Doc, here, figured it out."

Pleased that this visit had such a surprising, and positive, outcome, Dr. Vest added, "It was just common sense, the sort of thing that can't be learned from a book. While the cat was asleep, the feeding tube slid right down his esophagus. So I suspected that when he was awake and trying to eat, bits of food would hit the dangling object, pulling on the string looped under his tongue. That's what caused him to gag."

Tenderly petting the drowsy kitten, Natty glanced over to Nick, "At least you didn't have to follow Scrapper around in the middle of night with a flashlight, checking his litter box for buried treasure."

"We never thought of that," responded the coach. "It didn't occur to us that the missing diamond was *inside* Scrapper." Then, proudly, he held up the gem for all to see.

My partner and Coach Turner shook hands on their success. Then, unable to resist, Rich asked "May I?" as he reached for Nick's yard whistle and blew on it. The shrill pitch was enough to ignite barking from every dog in the kennel—signaling a celebration, of sorts.

For a vet, it's the measure of a day when it can end on a happy note. And, for Dr. Vest, this was one of those fine days.

Dirt Poor

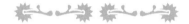

I knew Hoss O'Brien better than he knew himself. The feedlot farmer, who seemed unable to pull himself up from the depths of poverty, had called the clinic to report a problem with his cattle. And I could guess what was coming.

"My cows don't look so good, Doc...they've been losin' weight."

I had a bunch of questions, but, having known him for years, I already knew what his answers would be. "Have you wormed 'em lately?"

"Nope."

"Have you vaccinated 'em?"

"Nope."

"Have you watered 'em?"

"Yeah, they gotta whole tank of water."

"But, Hoss...have you checked it in the last month or two?"

When there was no answer, I asked again, "Well, have you?" I was always straight with him. And, by now, he also knew I'd never put up with his usual lame excuses.

So he, too, was frank. "Nope, Doc...my water pump broke."

Hoss was what some folks referred to as part of a 'backwoods clan'. After dropping out of school when he was only thirteen, he went into a self-imposed isolation by moving deep into the thick-forested area on the outskirts of town. He'd made it known that he didn't like people, and he didn't want anything to do with anyone in his own family, either. He lived in solitude during his teen years, but eventually managed to marry and start a family. Rarely venturing into town, he ended up keeping his wife and kids in seclusion, as well.

A large man, well over six feet tall, Hoss was mentally slow. I assumed he stayed away from people most of the time because it was just too difficult for him to cope.

Folks in town were wary of him. But, in spite of any faults or emotional problems he may have had, he was an honest lad. And, for some reason, he had an easy time with me. Maybe it was because I treated him just as fairly as I would any other client.

"What are you feeding your cows now, Hoss?"

After a long pause, he said, "I giv'd 'em some hay last week."

By this time, Dr. Vest had overheard some of the conversation. Sidling up to me, he poked me in the ribs to remind me that Hoss had a long overdue bill with us. So I asked, "Hoss, have you paid us yet for that calf delivery last winter?"

He laughed a little, and said, "I'll have ya some cash when y'all come out here, Doc."

So I teased him, "Cash, you've got cash? Well, then... I'll be right out to see you."

Tracy put her hands on her hips, like she always does when she's scolding me, "I hope you get paid this time...but I ain't holdin' my breath."

★ ★ ★ ★ ★

It was a hot, sticky hour's drive out to the O'Brien homestead. As soon as I got there, I caught a glimpse of the herd. In one small lot, there were around sixty head of mixed-breed cows, calves, and steers—all emaciated. And there wasn't a green blade of grass in sight.

The place hadn't changed a bit. Half the fences were down. Trash bags were stacked high next to the front door, and every window had its screens either torn or broken off. A half-dozen ol' coon dogs were sleeping on the weed-choked driveway as I pulled up honking my horn. The poor skinny mutts looked like rails. Yawning and stretching, they each got up slowly and meandered off into the high brush.

I didn't spot O'Brien anywhere. So I checked out the cattle pens and hay more closely. Mud, manure, and trampled stems from a two-year-old hay bale covered the area. I honked again...and again.

As I pulled up around the house near the backyard, two of O'Brien's eleven kids stopped their wrestling long enough to wave at me. Margi, his wife, turned to yell "Howdy," but continued to hang up her wash on the drooping clothes line that stretched from a fence post clear across the yard. I'd often wondered about Margi, and felt that she didn't seem to fit out here. She'd gone through school in town and was headed to college when she met Hoss. Still quite attractive, the raven-haired woman had changed little over the years. She was always cheerful and patient. But, surprisingly, she never seemed tired, even though she'd been raising all these kids with no help at all.

From the shade under the porch's overhang came O'Brien's basso voice. "Hey, gringo...'bout time you got here. Damn'd cows coulda died by now. And what's all the noise 'bout...you ain't gotta honk."

Hoss didn't seem in any hurry to move from the comfort of his chair. After rubbing his hands over its threadbare arms, he grumbled and hoisted his 300-pound frame up and out of the seat. He towered over me. "Good to see ya, Doc. Like I said, the cows ain't been lookin' healthy for weeks. But, thanks for comin' out."

As usual, Hoss rarely wore shirts or socks. He just had on denim overalls, and, from the looks of them, they'd obviously missed Margi's last few washes. But he was careful enough to fetch his rubber boots next to the doorway, and pull them up over his shoeless feet.

While taking me through the potholed yard to the pens, he pointed out three cows standing away from the main herd. As we walked toward them, we passed four of his scantily clad boys, playing on a broken down, rusty truck. I didn't say anything about the $125 dollars he owed the clinic. But when we got to the pen's gate, he handed me twenty dollars and fourteen cents. At least he remembered—and, at least, something was better than nothing.

"Hoss, where did the cattle here come from?"

"South Texas," he proudly said, "...and got one hell of a deal, too."

After scanning the herd, it didn't take me long to realize he'd been 'taken'. But I wasn't going to tell him that the animals bore a Mexican brand. And the specific brand identified them as part of a larger group recently smuggled across the border. Clinics throughout the state receive fax alerts from the Department of Agriculture on a regular basis. So we'd been informed about a herd of five hundred, known to be sick even before they entered the United States.

The three depressed cows Hoss had pointed out were dying in a standing position. As I came up to the first, it was obvious she couldn't even walk anymore. The second had a look in her eye that said she was gone already. I asked Hoss to guide the third into his makeshift squeeze chute. As he did so, she weaved and stumbled from weakness. But, unthinking, he slammed the head gate as though she might escape. So I quickly grabbed her tail to keep her from collapsing. Long strings of drool were dripping from her pale yellow gums, and her horns hung down so low that they scraped the ground. There were ticks, lice, and flies trying to bite through her brown hide. This was a living, breathing skeleton with skin— and I wondered how I could possibly keep her alive.

I looked down at the water trough, but couldn't see the water due to the green algae floating in it. Now I knew why I was the only vet Hoss called upon. I reckoned the others were smarter than me and wouldn't put up with this type of situation. I was beginning to think I was a glutton for punishment—unpaid punishment, at that.

Pulling a corncob pipe from his pocket, Hoss lit up some tobacco that smelled worse than the cattle pens. Flies flew off with each puff of smoke. And the farmer said, "Whatdya think, Doc...is she sick?"

Since the cow could barely stand, his question shocked me. He either didn't know or care about what went on around him. The cow's breathing was labored, and her temperature was high. She showed about every negative symptom possible: dehydration, malnutrition, jaundice, diarrhea, lack of coordination and a reluctance to move.

"Does she have 'monia'?" asked Hoss.

After giving the cow a dose of dextrose and the antibiotic oxytetracycline, I drew blood from her jugular vein for lab analysis. As I checked each animal, I saw that even the healthiest were showing symptoms of a disease. "No, it's not pneumonia, Hoss...but your whole herd is infected."

"With what?"

"I'm not sure yet. That's why I'm collecting these random samples of blood. I'll call you when the results come back. Then we'll know how to proceed."

Glad to get back into Ol' Blue for my trip home, I said my goodbyes and turned the ignition key. But the truck just sputtered on empty. "Hoss, I didn't realize I was running so low...do you have any fuel?"

"Sure, Doc," grinned the big guy.

Returning to Dallas, I walked into Meadow Creek and handed Rachel my fourteen cents in change...all that was left after 'paying' for my gas at the O'Brien place.

When the lab reports came back, they confirmed my worst suspicions. The O'Brien's cattle had anaplasmosis. Seeing the look on my face after I called Hoss to tell him, Tracy was anxious to know more about the disease. But as I began to tell her, Dr. Vest made an announcement, "Tracy, get me all the oxytetracycline you can locate. And Rachel, call Hoss and tell him I'm comin' out there this time. Doc, you stay here...you're too soft on those folks. I'll treat the herd, fix the water pump...*and* I'll get us paid once and for all."

* * * * *

After honking and yelling, my partner heard Margi's voice hollering out from the back porch, "Come 'round back, Doc. Can ya fix our cows now?" With two scrawny girls clinging to her long, handmade skirt, Mrs. O'Brien came down the back steps wiping her hands on a wrap-around towel apron.

Pointing beyond the yard to where the older kids were playing, she said, "Hoss is over yonder. Come on, you can follow me."

Rich followed Margi's barefooted prints in the wet dirt trail. Apparently, there was only one set of rubber boots in the family...and everyone took turns. As Rich viewed the surroundings, Margi asked, "Doctor Vest, are our cows as sick as Doc Carlton thought they were?"

Responding with a brief "Yeah, they are," Rich kept staring at the smallest child's face. He couldn't take his eyes away from the apparent sadness. Her cheeks were smudged with mud, and her dress was patched, though clean. Margi must have quickly dressed her when she heard Rich honking. Holding a little unclothed doll close to her chest, 'Eleven' —as she was called—looked up at Rich with bewitching hazel eyes. But she never smiled.

When he reached the gate, Dr. Vest waited for Hoss to see him. He could already smell the strong tobacco, as well as the odor coming from the mold in the water tank. Then he saw the three cows I'd described to him still standing by themselves apart from the rest. Hoss turned just as one of the boys bolted out of the house, jumped the steps, and shouted, "Are you the vet?"

George was the O'Brien's third eldest child—or 'Three' as Hoss would say, since he rarely remembered his children's names. George was out of breath, but his eyes were gleaming. And my partner sensed that the tall, gangly boy, who could be around twelve, was very different from his father. The boy held up a thick book, then began flipping through the pages excitedly saying, "I know all about ana-plas-mo-sis. Read it right here on page 269. See?" None of the kids went to school, so Rich guessed that Margi must have taught him to read.

Hoss interrupted the boy, "Now, you hush, Three, and let the doctor do the talkin'. Don't mind his foolishness, Doc. All he does is dream. He's always with the animals or readin'. Can't get no work out of 'im. So don't 'spect he'll amount to much."

"But, Pa...please..."

"Hush, now...I said."

George reluctantly obeyed his papa. But Rich couldn't disregard the boy's eagerness. Overlooking Hoss' objections, my partner took a few minutes to encourage George's interest by joining him in perusing the pages of his book on animal husbandry. It startled him, though, to see that this was a relatively new and expensive book with the latest information. There were no libraries out here in the woods. So he was going to ask the boy about it, when Margi pulled on his sleeve urging him to tell them what was happening with their cattle.

Summoning up his resolve, and pulling no punches, Dr. Vest began, "Mr. and Mrs. O'Brien, the way I see it, we have three big problems. Y'all have very sick cattle with a serious disease...and there's a real expense in treating that disease. But, even if they survive after treatment, there's no way they can be healthy again unless you give them fresh water *every* day, and fresh hay *every* day. If you can't do that, we might as well let them die right here, right now."

After a full minute or two of silence, Margi reached deep down into her skirt pocket and brought out a small coin purse. But Hoss put up his hand, saying, "Whoa, now...we're gonna talk about this."

But Margi had already made up her mind and was determined to follow through. Fumbling with her change and counting it, she emptied the purse into the palm of her hand and held it out to Dr. Vest. "I think there's twenty-three dollars here. It's just a beginning...but take it, Doc...and God bless ya."

"Now, Doc...tell us true...what's this ana-stuff?" asked Hoss.

Finding himself at a loss for words, my partner's plan to remain firm dissolved. He stood there in front of the whole barefooted O'Brien clan, holding most of their life savings.

Clearing his throat, he answered the farmer's question as thoroughly as possible. "This disease can be called anaplasmosis or gall sickness. It's caused by a rickettsia organism, which we can call the 'R' bug. It brings on anemia and icterus."

He stopped briefly to wink at the little girl with the naked doll, who blushed and tried to wink back...using both eyes.

"Anyway, the RBCs are infected and destroyed, and the hepatic and spleen congestion..." Stopping himself from going on, Dr. Vest knew that George was the only one who could understand him. So he simply said, "Hoss, they get poor blood, run high fevers, quit eating and drinking, turn yellow from bad livers...and die."

"But where does it come from?" Hoss asked.

"It's spread from animal to animal by direct mechanical transmission."

Looking confused, Hoss said, "But, Doc, my pickup ain't been runnin' lately."

Smiling patiently, Rich said, "No, Hoss...it's not that kind of mechanics. The 'R' bug is spread by direct blood transfer from biting flies or ticks...or the use of a common needle."

Looking over at her husband with a frown, Margi said, "Lord knows, we got plenty of them flies. I've been complainin' to Hoss 'bout it for a long while." The farmer wasn't going to take a lecture from a woman in front of another man...so he turned and began banging his pipe on the fence post.

"Folks, we'll need to treat your cattle every day. Keep them up in the evenings and have them ready to be injected. Doc Carlton, Dr. Horton and I will take turns comin' by. Now, let's get started."

"C'mon boys," Hoss yelled, "Y'all come help me and the doctor now...and, girls, y'all go back to the house with your ma."

"Just a second," said Rich, as he knelt down next to the five-year-old with the doll. Pulling out all the money he'd just received from Margi, he stuffed it into the round pockets of her dress. "Here, sweetheart, you give this to your mama, okay?" Then, reaching for his wallet, he took out another five-dollar bill. "And, this here...is just for you and your doll."

* * * * *

Rich strolled into the clinic, trying to avoid the knowing glances from Tracy and Rachel who stood there defiantly. "Well, how did it go, Doctor V...did ya get our bill paid?" asked Tracy.

"It went well," mumbled Rich, handing over his last dollar bill, while the staff tried to suppress giggling.

"You and your big speeches, you're even more of a softie than Doc, here," chastised Rachel.

"And how are the cattle doing?" I asked.

"They're better, Doc...I think they'll all make it providing the family makes some changes. You can go out tomorrow, then Natty and I will take turns after that. By the way, have you met George? I told him and his folks that we've made him our 'Veterinary Assistant in Training'. And he's to call us whenever there's a medical question.

"I also took him aside and told him to be responsible for the daily watering and feeding of the herd. He's going to take the dogs under his wing, too, and provide them with the dog chow I gave him. And since these assignments will be supervised by us, Hoss won't give the boy any trouble."

"Yep...he's a sharp kid." I said. "We'll be seeing a lot more of him. I also have a feeling he'd make a good vet."

Rich went on praising George, "He has all the right symptoms, doesn't he? He's just like we were at that age. Hell, that boy's so broke...but he doesn't seem to let it bother him. Under our tutoring, he'll work on his pa's animals for free. And that'll eventually save us time and money, too."

Then, deciding to give me a bad time, he said, "By they way, have you seen that latest medical volume we ordered last year? It's missing from our research shelf. You don't suppose some mushy-hearted vet gave it away, do you?"

"So, you got me." I laughed, "But we both feel that we'll see George O'Brien with a D.V.M. behind his name one day. Nothing would please us more, right? And anything we can do to make it happen is worth it."

Always the sensitive observer, Rich was quiet for a moment, then said, "Why do you suppose there's so little middle ground in our business? Have you noticed that we either serve the super-wealthy folks with multi-million dollar ranches—or the dirt-poor farmers who go from day to day barely managing to survive. Is that just the way it is in Texas—a land of extremes—with either the very rich or the very poor?"

I rarely debated Rich or even pondered on such broad social issues. Quite simply, all I knew was that we'd just adopted ourselves a new family. Something good came from something bad. And that's just the way it was.

15

Sidekick

Almost every day, after springing into the passenger seat of Ol' Blue, my pal would be ready for 'take off'. And all I had to say was "C'mon, Aggie." This canine was fast becoming my constant companion as I took to the road covering calls throughout the north of Dallas. Her poky littermate, Lugar, on the other hand, was a stay-at-home. The two rottweilers couldn't have been more different. While Aggie brimmed with energy and curiosity, her brother sleepily looked on, preferring to move as little as possible. Even during the few times when Lugar came along, he'd use the trips to catch up on more snoozing.

Normally, Tracy would accompany me. But since we were still short on staff, her valuable medical expertise was now needed by Dr. Vest at Meadow Creek. So, it was Aggie who left with me at dawn to travel from stable to stable and farm to farm. Though I missed gabbing with Tracy, this temporary arrangement was becoming fun, especially since my dog was the only one who didn't whine about the bumpy rides in my old truck.

This spirited pooch thrived on road adventures. As soon as I'd close the cab door and roll down the window, her whole body would tense with anticipation. And her haughty, erect posture left no question as to who was 'in charge'. She'd hold her chest out proudly, while keeping her front paws perched on the window's edge. And as Ol' Blue flew along the freeways, my eager pup seemed to be in 'dog heaven'... squinting her eyelids and thrusting her nose way up into the winds, letting the gusts blow at her face and flap her ears around. I imagined that if she could talk, she'd say, *"Look at me...I'm flying."*

Her spontaneous reactions to every happening were so entertaining that I promised myself to continue bringing her along, even after Tracy joined me again. But since I was so accustomed to discussing cases with my assistant as we drove, I found myself doing the same with Aggie—as if she could understand every word.

After one such call from Cathy Radcliff, I announced, "Well, girl, we're headed out to see Cathy now." After a muffled bark, Aggie wiggled in her seat and her nubbed tail wagged furiously. "Okay, okay...I'll hurry. You remember Miss Radcliff. She's that nice teller at my bank's drive-up window... the one who leaves you a dog biscuit in the canister whenever we make our clinic's deposits. She's crazy about horses...but taking care of them keeps her broke."

We made a quick stop at the bank, but Aggie became restless when there was no sign of Cathy or her treat. "I forgot to tell you, we're meeting your friend at the new stable."

I'd been surprised when Cathy told me she'd bought another horse. She could barely afford her bills now. But the jovial, robust lady was so warm-hearted that she couldn't resist adopting an animal in need. Unfortunately, she was now known as a 'barn jumper'. This was the fourth time in a year she'd been asked to leave a location because she couldn't always pay the stall rent on time.

It was a good thing I remembered to ask her where the horses were stabled now, or I'd have ended up in the wrong place. She'd called asking help for her latest addition, Boss Man, who had a cut lip. "There's a new barn on the backside of the Milper homestead, between the Lazy Z stable and the ol' Shiloh place," she said. "Look for the fresh white-shell road and the large wooden mailbox carved to look like a life-sized rooster. I'll be waiting at the top of the rise."

I knew the vicinity and headed toward the new spot. There was only one rooster-shaped postbox on Jupiter Road, right under a neon sign that blinked *EAT MORE BEEF* in rotating colors of green, orange and yellow. "We're at the right place now, Aggie."

Spotting Miss Radcliff before I did, Aggie just about jumped out of her seat. Her black ears perked straight up, and she couldn't stop barking. She adored this woman, and the feeling was mutual.

I pulled up and reached over Aggie to push open the side door. "Howdy, Cathy...climb in and we'll go check on Boss Man."

My big black dog had an instinctive and accurate ability to judge character. And she turned to mush around this sweet lady, continually licking her cheeks while Cathy tried to climb into the seat. "Scoot over, girl," she giggled, "and let me in."

"Aggie, quit givin' kisses," I said, "and try to sit still."

With Cathy pointing the way, we headed toward a modern, orange-metal barn in the middle of a tranquil meadow. Hidden away from the surrounding noises of the expressway, this architecturally designed T-shaped stable and equine center was a new addition to the area. Its sprawling office and barn-compound had a half-dozen stalls lined up on each side. And a long indoor arena became the main body of the 'T' layout. Next to the circular drive, two small boys with their parents were petting a black and white pony in a round corral. Responding to their squeals of delight, Aggie bounced up and down at the window when one of the boys waved at her.

The barn's entranceway was flanked by tall adobe pots of freshly planted pansies and geraniums. And grazing in the grassy pasture next to the structure were the stable's many steeds—with Cathy's five other horses among them.

Just as I commented, "This is a pretty uptown place," a white limousine pulled into the drive. The chauffeur quickly jumped out to open the trunk, carefully lifting out what looked to be a brand new saddle. The limo's occupants, a lovely blond girl and a mid-aged gent, wearing a dark, ill-fitting hairpiece, watched the driver closely and seemed to be ordering him about.

"There's Mr. Gilbert," Cathy said, "He's letting me use one of the maintenance sheds for a stall. Instead of rent, all I have to do is vacuum his office once a week, and feed his horses every evening." Something about this arrangement bothered me, but I didn't say anything.

Cathy called out a greeting to the man as we slowly coasted by on the path leading to the back of the snazzy barn. Unseen behind the new building were some old tool sheds… or, more accurately, temporary lean-tos.

"Here we are, Doc…and there's Boss Man." I was eager to take a look at her horse. Unexpectedly, Aggie began growling and her neck muscles were rigid. We couldn't figure out what was bothering her. Then, over our shoulder, we saw the stable's owner striding up the path with his lady friend.

He hollered over to me, "I'm Bill Gilbert…and you must be Doc Carlton." Reaching my side, he vigorously extended his arm, and we shook hands.

I took a glance at Aggie and got more than a little concerned. Her low, ominous growl turned into a snarl, and her lips curled back over her teeth. "Aggie, lay down, now!" I ordered. Well-trained, she obeyed, but kept up her raspy growling.

As Cathy began to tell me more about her colt, Bill Gilbert interrupted, "I've got a couple of *good* horses I want you to look at first."

I ignored his attitude, while trying to remain courteous. "Sure, be glad to...when I'm done with Boss Man here."

Cathy again started to discuss her horse's injury, when Bill loudly proclaimed, "Miss Radcliff, your horse can wait. I want Doc to see my horses and Julie's mare, Brassy, who turned up lame this mornin'. Right now, Doc!" With that, he grabbed at my jacket. I prayed that Aggie didn't see this as I swiftly pulled my sleeve from his grasp. But when I stood there looking at him straight on...I began to notice that something was not quite right.

The arrogant fellow, about fifty, was desperately trying to look twenty. He stood there in blue linen trousers and a blue silk shirt, left unbuttoned and wide open over his bare chest. Several strands of gold chains hung from his neck to his navel. And, in his high-heeled lizard boots, he even managed to add three inches to his height. The nineteen- or twenty-year-old woman on his arm never spoke...but just kept gazing at him with awe.

This time, when Cathy tried to tell me that Boss Man had cut his lip on a nail in that shed she was renting, I quietly said, "Bill, I'll be looking at Miss Radcliff's horse *first*."

Obviously put out, especially since he liked showing off in front of his girlfriend, the fellow nonetheless backed down, saying, "Well, if you need my help, me and Julie will be in *my* brand new, high-tech office." He pulled the girl close to him and whispered in her ear. She giggled when he seductively said, "This'll give us some time to ourselves, Sugar...and you know I can tame most anything."

Aggie quieted down as soon as the couple left. I even considered putting her in the truck, since I wasn't sure how she'd react if the braggart came back again. But I decided to wait. I wanted to see Boss Man right away, since Cathy mentioned how skittish he was. And the ruckus in front of his stall didn't help any.

A good-looking red roan, the colt was a long-yearling Appaloosa with a splattering of white dapples on his rump. And he was big for his age. When he spun his body around to face me, I saw the fear in his eyes. So I spoke softly, "Whoa, boy." But I'd been leaning against a rickety plank fence, and it suddenly creaked as one of the boards snapped. Already wound up, Boss Man spooked, whirled and kicked the wall. This wasn't going to be easy. The horse had a four-inch tear in the flesh of his jaw. And he'd never been haltered. At 700 pounds, he was too strong to handle and too frightened to stand still. I looked over to Cathy, nodded, and crawled through the fence toward the horse.

Figuring that total patience was our only hope with this youngster, I coaxed, "Whoa, boy, whoa," and lightly touched Boss Man on the neck. His muscles flinched. "Cathy, hand me the extra-large halter," I said. My knees were shaking, but I went on crooning to him in a calm, steady voice. Sweat ran down my back, and I kept the halter hidden until I stepped into the right position. Then, in one delicate move, I slid the soft nylon harness around his neck, and slipped the bridle strap over his muzzle. Though he tensed and snorted, he didn't erupt. But I wasn't fool enough to think he wouldn't try. If anything touched the raw issue on his jaw, he'd explode. I whispered, "Easy, boy...no one's going to hurt you." After the loose-fitting halter glided over the bridge of his nose, I finally sighed. "See? That's all there is to it." Hooking the clasp and patting him, I reached in my pocket for the already prepared tranquilizer. I still needed to inject his vein and stitch the wound. The prick of the needle didn't seem to bother the young horse. So far, so good...I thought. "Now, boy...you can relax for a while...we're halfway there."

Just then, my dog streaked by us in a barking frenzy. Bill Gilbert was bellowing, "Doc, aren't you done yet?" I quickly turned, but the commotion startled Boss Man again. And my efforts to calm him were undone. Something struck me above the eye, and I felt the horse's hoof hitting my shoulder as I fell against the top board rails of the stall. In the blur of the moment, I could hear Bill's voice. And Cathy was screaming at him. He was grabbing and jerking Boss Man's lead rope.

Scrambling to get up on my feet, I yelled, "Wait! Don't do that!" But the son-of-a...began thrashing a buggy whip across the chest and loins of the tranquilized, defenseless colt.

WHAP–WHAP. "Damn you!" he swore at the horse. "I'll show you who's the boss around here!" WHAP–WHAP–WHAP.

"Doc, stop him!" Cathy cried.

Instinctively, I called out, "Aggie...git him!" My husky rottweiler was at my side in a flash, snarling. And it took all my strength to hold her back from lunging at him. "Not one more blow from you, Bill!" I shouted. There was a proverbial line drawn in the sand...and he'd just crossed it.

"You've gotta show these animals who's boss...and that's what I intend to do," he said.

"Try it again and let's see how Aggie here feels about it. Or, you can drop that whip in the dirt—right now!" I loosened my grip a little on Aggie's leash, and her sudden thrust toward the abusive fellow was enough to make him let go of the whip, and release the colt's lead rope.

Mumbling, "Oh, suit yourself, Doc," Gilbert slowly turned and walked up the path, glancing over his shoulder every few seconds to see if Aggie was coming after him.

Bringing me a towel for the cut over my eyebrow, Cathy bent down to congratulate my heroic dog, "Aggie, girl...ya done good." Proud of herself, and acting like she'd fended off a mortal enemy, Aggie rolled over on her back and let Cathy stroke her tummy.

Apparently, nothing during this emotionally charged incident was lost on Boss Man. Critters often have a mysterious way of understanding more than we realize. Now that calm was restored, the high-strung horse whinnied, and came forward to nudge my arm. After I blotted and medicated the whip marks, I examined his jaw wound. And Cathy held his lead rope while I sewed eight sutures to close the skin. Always comfortable around horses, Aggie went up to Boss Man and stood in front of him...looking up at the tall animal like she was waiting for something. The colt then lowered his neck and touched his nose to hers. This was a common occurrence with Aggie, and I never got tired of seeing it.

"That Gilbert fellow may have given you this location, Cathy, but your horse shouldn't suffer for it. The man will continue pulling these power plays. You need to move your horses to a decent place. I don't think he'll mess with Boss Man again. But that doesn't mean he won't try something with your other horses."

Though still shaken, Cathy asked, "In spite of what happened, I'd like to watch you examine Bill's horses. Besides, I could really use you there for moral support when I give him notice that I won't be working for him anymore."

"Sure...however, I'm only doing this brief exam for him once. But let's leave the truck parked here and walk over to the pasture." I knew we needed to have Aggie wait in the cab, out of sight, because I just wasn't sure what would happen if she came anywhere near Bill again.

"Are you ready, Cathy? This may be more fun than you think. So, let's go take him on!"

But our last one-on-one meeting with the abrasive stable owner was less like fun...and more like a quick and quiet getaway. Uttering as few words as possible, I checked his horses, told him they were fine and handed him the name of another vet. Then Cathy summoned up courage to deliver her speech, which was short, frank and honest. Bill nodded, and said nothing. In fact, he didn't even raise his eyes to look at either one of us.

But as we were about to leave, Julie came out of the arena leading a gentle brown and white Paint mare. I was surprised when she asked me why Brassy had turned lame. It was the first time she'd spoken up...and she was very sweet. So I took the time to examine her docile animal.

But Bill chimed in, "Look, I know he's got Summer sore. And I already told you, Julie, that's why he's lame."

"No, that's *not* the reason," I said. "Summer sores or Jack sores are fairly typical, and show up as skin diseases. There are several stages in the progression. But the point of origin emanates from stable flies. These few lesions can be treated, but may heal slowly."

Abruptly, he asked, "So...is this goin' to cost me a damn fortune? And if it's not the sore, then why in the hell is she limping on her left front leg?"

I now wanted to speak slowly and clearly so Julie would understand every word. "She's not lame on the left. Brassy's lame on her *right* front...because you bowed her tendon."

Arguing, Bill said, "Aw, c'mon now...I didn't ride her hard."

This was the opening Cathy and I were waiting for. What he'd done to Boss Man would have its price. This time I spoke loudly, "Brassy's bowed tendon is the result of all *your* whip welts on her rear!"

"Whip marks!" screamed Julie. "You beat Brassy?" Stunned for a second, the little lady showed backbone after all. She pounded her fists against Bill's chest, calling him every name under the sun. Cathy and I made a swift exit while Julie continued yelling at the top of her lungs. A few minutes later, we were back in the truck rolling out of the compound. As we pulled around past the pasture gate, we saw that Julie had grabbed the buggy whip and was running after Bill, wildly waving the whip with intent to use it on him. We didn't need to stay and watch. Besides, when Aggie saw all this, she went absolutely nuts...and Cathy needed to restrain her or she would have bolted through the window to join Julie in the chase.

I'd barely finished relaying the day's events to my partner, when—always trumping me—he immediately laid out a plan for Cathy. As luck would have it, Dr. Vest's cousin, Jason, had a small spread in the north. Lately, he'd been complaining to Rich that after his daughter married, she moved her horses to Colorado. Since then, Jason and his wife have had the 'empty nest' doldrums. And they missed the horses almost as much as they missed their daughter. So when Rich told them about Cathy, they could hardly wait to ask her to bring Boss Man and the rest of her small equine herd out to their place...rent free.

Best of all, Aggie is always ready and waiting to hit the trails again. I wouldn't think of taking on the world without her.

16

Strange Bonds

hil Eastman's training facility in Roanoke managed three hundred cutting horses. And it was probably the best place for our newest colleague to get broken in. But for three nights running—at midnight, to be precise—Phil called him out to treat his Quarter horse gelding for a sudden onset of muscle spasms.

These late night ranch visits lasted well until 3:00 A.M... and by Friday, Dr. Horton was dragging. So Dr. Vest and I decided to treat him to some end-of-the-week 'downtime' at a nearby pub. The Bunkhouse Saloon had been a longtime watering hole for the area's overworked blue-collar folks. Its new managers, however, decided to fancy-it-up for tourists by remodeling it into their concept of an upscale western tavern with light oak furniture, polished brass rails and fittings, and hand-painted French floor tiles.

Slowly tagging after one another, we made our way in through the dimly lit atmosphere, and headed past starched cloth-covered tables toward the long drover's bar. The three of us were dead tired. Rich propped his elbows on the antique bar's surface, and locked one of his boot heels over the foot rail. We each did the same...in turn. Natty hadn't said anything on the way in. And, still quiet, he held up three fingers for his order.

There, standing in front of us, was the saloon's original innkeeper, Mavis Rhodes. It was good to see the tough ol' gal...and it was also a surprise to see her. The managers, whom she had hired before her retirement, told her they were bringing in cute young gals in western garb as waitresses. It didn't work; the tourists didn't come. If this place on Commerce Street were to have any business at all, they'd have to bring back Mavis—the one person who made the place 'home' to the locals.

"Howdy, Docs...what'll ya have?" she asked loudly. Behind her was one of the gaudy 1906 naked-lady paintings from her original bar. She'd retrieved it from the storeroom and hastily hung it up over the newly imported wine racks.

Thumbing his hat back, Rich half-mumbled, "Gimme three longnecks, Mavis...and how are ya, gal?"

Yanking the perennial towel off from her shoulder, she wiped up a client's spilled beer, and, in her inimitable scratchy voice, said, "Aw...Rich, wouldn't do no good to complain. My arthritis is actin' up a bit. But, other than that...well...you know how it goes."

Even after thirty years, Mavis loved her job. The matron's blond curly hair, often brown at the roots, gave her a frazzled look. But she had an ear for news and she never forgot a thing. After listening to the woes of many, she still had so much compassion that some called her 'Mother Mavis'. Her finely tuned intuition could spot even the subtlest of problems. She'd inherited the popular gathering spot after her husband died of liver failure...an unfortunate, but common, malady among barkeeps. I'd always marveled that there didn't seem to be anyone in Dallas, or in several counties around, that Mavis didn't know.

With an expert hand, she slid three longnecks down the thirty-foot stretch of mahogany. Each one made a smooth swishing sound as it went gliding over the highly waxed surface.

After a few long draws on his bottle, Rich poked Natty and asked, "Now, tell us what's been happening at Phil's place...and what's bothering his favorite horse? I heard ya came up with some secret cure."

We were well acquainted with the clinical signs of 'azoturia'. Both Rich and I had seen our share of performance horses on high protein food. Hobbled by infrequent exercise programs, they ended up suffering from heavy sweating, nervous tremors, and a reluctance to move. My last case with a three-year-old thoroughbred had started out with a mild stiffness in the hindquarters. The condition spread so rapidly that the horse was reduced to a mass of twitching muscles before finally responding to treatments.

After slinging the wet towel back across her shoulder, Mavis dried her hands on an apron that only slightly covered her plumpish-round tummy. Then folding her bare arms across her breasts, she targeted Dr. Horton. "Natty...you gotta long face tonight. But glad to see you can still prop yourself up at my bar. What's ailin' ya, son?"

If anyone could get Natty Horton to talk, it would be Mavis. Taking a short swig of brew and setting the frosty bottle back down, our boy honestly said, "I don't rightly know."

A slight smile crossed Mavis's unpainted lips, then spread across her kind face. Turning to me, she said, "Whelp, it's gotta be a woman or a horse. Nothin' else could put that scowl on a young man's brow." Her fingers tapped on the ashtray she'd just cleaned. And as one of the gents at the counter left, she reached for his empty glass and stuffed the buck tip down into the cleavage of her red sleeveless blouse. Continuing to prod, she asked, "Who is she, Natty?"

At that, our colleague shyly opened up. "Remember Phil Eastman? Well, he's got this gelding that..."

The crusty gal's smile broadened. "Do you mean that bay cutter who glides like a duck on water, Justice for All? The one with freckles on his right flank and the two white socks on his forelegs?" Shaking our heads in wonderment, Rich and I just looked at one another. Mavis really did know everything.

As she repositioned one of her dangling gold earrings, Mavis gave Natty a sly look, "Well, I already told you 'bout Scat."

Natty quickly put his finger up to his lips indicating he wanted her to hush up.

"Scat?" Dr. Vest asked, "Who's Scat?"

"I think Scat's the cat." I offered. "And is that what all this is about?"

My partner slapped his hands on his knees, "Will somebody here please tell me what Mavis knows and what Dr. Horton won't talk about?"

"Aw, Mavis, you weren't going to say anything," complained Natty.

"I speak my mind, even when it ain't been asked for. And, y'all can't say I'm wrong," laughed Mavis.

After handing Dr. Horton another beer 'on the house', Mavis added, "Look, son, the answer's been Scat all along."

"Natty, what's she hinting at?" asked Rich.

Since she'd pulled no punches, Mavis had cracked Dr. Horton's veneer. Our super-efficient doctor of medicine didn't really want to admit to Dr. Vest or me that a mangy ol' barn cat could fix what he couldn't—or that Mavis was the one to help him solve Justice for All's on-and-off illness. Finally grinning, Natty winked at Mavis as she was buffing up another spill on the counter. "You know, gal..you're gonna wear a hole in that wood."

"And I know you're changin' the subject, boy. Now, tell us all 'bout Scat. The last time I saw him, he was too wild for anyone to get near him."

While flipping a pretzel back and forth from one hand to the other, Natty haltingly said, "I...caught him...and he and I came to a mutual agreement..."

"Now we're getting somewhere...I gotta hear this," said Rich, as he moved closer to the bar.

"Okay, here it is. Every night out at the Circle L was pretty much the same. There'd been no rain. So the barn aisles were moist and slick from the usual low-slung fog and humidity. You've been there...and you know that fog is knee high. It was late, and the horses were all in their stalls. But I couldn't even see their hooves. Snorts and whinnies greeted me and echoed throughout the quiet winter night. The fuss was loud enough to let Phil know I'd arrived, and it usually took him about five minutes to show up. My boots would be wet, and my face was always cold. I could see my own breaths in front of me. Being there alone felt eerie. The stalls' wooden sides seemed to sweat as droplets of moisture dripped from the metal rafters above them.

"The trainer, hunched over with frustration, would come in looking so worried about his gelding that he'd hardly give me a glance. And, each night, he'd say the same thing, 'Dr. Horton, he's doin' it again.'"

As he took another sip of brew, Natty looked from me to Rich to Mavis and went on. "You know, Justice had the same symptoms for three straight nights—for no apparent reason. This horse is normally as fit and muscular as any animal could be. And Phil has a heat lamp over his stall... so the horse's back is kept warm as toast."

"So...what was going on?" Rich asked.

"He'd be sweating profusely, hyperventilating, cramping, and his loin muscles were stiff. He didn't even want to move."

Turning to me, Rich said, "Sounds like an open and shut case to me. Must be azoturia, or Monday morning illness as we call it now."

"That's right," Natty agreed, "...but psycho-induced? Phil told me that Justice for All is fine all day long. Then, around 9:00 P.M., his behavior changes...and he becomes very erratic. He begins by pacing up and down. Then he works himself up into a frenetic lather until his muscles actually freeze up."

Both Dr. Vest and I repeated the same thing, "No, that's not possible. A condition such as azoturia just doesn't come and go."

This was all very strange. And we could now see why Natty had been so baffled. Monday morning disease was difficult enough to diagnose, but the 'why' of it was even harder...especially in this case, since the onset appeared very late in the evening...and at the same time every night.

"I was so frustrated by this *Twilight Zone* type of scenario," Natty said, "that I found myself mulling it over with Mavis after I'd treated Justice for the third time with anti-inflammatory therapy. I knew there was some missing link between physical exercise, food rations, and maybe an emotional trigger. Though the exercise arena was too wet for a workout, I still had Phil jog the gelding up and down the barn aisle. I reduced his high-protein diet and supplemented it with Vitamin E and selenium. I wanted to rule out the quality and quantity of grain and hay as a possible factor. Justice has a good life. Phil couldn't be taking better care of him. So what was I overlooking?

"That's when Mavis here told me it all made perfect sense to her, when she unexpectedly asked me, 'Where was the cat during those three nights?'"

Dr. Horton looked over at the perceptive woman and, in exasperation, said, "Mavis, now could you please tell the good doctors what you told me?"

This time, Mavis drew a draft for herself and leaned back to fill in the details for the missing puzzle piece. "When I spotted Dr. Horton come through those swinging doors a couple night ago, he was still wearin' the same brown shirt he'd worn the night before. His boots were muddy, the brim of his hat hung low, and he shuffled his feet like a man carryin' a heavy burden."

"Mavis...Mavis...," interrupted Rich, "...forget the drama, and just tell us about the cat."

Striking a match to relight her cigarette, Mavis went on, "Scat's his name. He's a scraggly ol' tomcat...and as wild as a March hare. He's all yellow...tall and scrawny...and he ain't got but part of one ear. No tellin' how many fights he's had."

She inhaled deeply and blew a perfect smoke ring. It floated above her head and rested there like a halo.

"Well, during the time when I was tryin' to catch Phil's eye…'cause it ain't no secret that I've had a crush on him for years…I'd go out to the Circle L to watch him ride as he prepped his horses for competition. Then, afterwards, the two of us would stroll through the barns. That's when I first saw him."

"Who?"we asked in unison.

"Scat, the cat," Mavis snapped. "Pay attention, now." Another silver ring of smoke billowed forth. And the music got louder as several patrons took up boot-scootin' in the corner near the jukebox.

"Anyway, I watched Justice for All raise his head while lookin' up for Scat. And from high up in the rafters, the cat would appear. He'd crawl across the narrowest rail, then jump onto a post, where—like a fireman—he would slither and slide all the way down to the floor. I was amazed by his acrobatics. Then he'd wait by the feed bin. When Justice came close enough, he'd leap onto the horse and snuggle himself into a comfortable ball right in the center of Justice's back. And that's where he slept all night…getting full benefit from the warmth of the horse's heat lamp. When Phil saw me watching this, he nonchalantly told me that the two were buddies. But I never figured the horse would go into a frenzy until the other night, when Natty told me about the problem."

Draining his beer with a final gulp, Rich said, "I'll be damned. You're telling me that a yellow cat caused Justice for All to have a psychosomatic illness?"

"No," Natty said, "She's telling you that the *loss* of the cat caused Justice's emotional trauma."

"Animals can form bonds that are stronger than any medicine," I added. "For months, Scat has crawled onto Justice's back at bedtime. But when he went cattin' around and failed to show up for three nights in a row, the sorrel gelding went into a tizzy."

Dr. Vest jumped up, reeled on his heels and headed toward the saloon's open doors, "Let's go...I've gotta see this for myself!" Mavis yelled to her staff that she was going, too.

Rich and Natty took off in Ol' Blue, while Mavis and I followed in her red Mustang. Twenty minutes later, we pulled into the Circle L Ranch, and jumped out. The figure of Phil Eastman came out from the swirling fog that was blanketing the barn door. Shading his eyes from our headlights, he motioned for us to come inside while asking, "What are y'all doin' here tonight? And Mavis, is that you?"

I'm sure we looked like four rowdies out on the town, so I briefly explained ourselves. "Phil, we just heard about this unusual situation and had to see it for ourselves. How's Justice for All doing?"

Pointing to a quiet stall, he said, "See for yourself, Doc. Thanks to all that Dr. Horton did, I have a feeling my gelding has a chance to win the Futurity Cuttin' in two weeks at the Fort Worth coliseum."

Justice for All was the perfect picture of tranquility and serenity. He moved with ease and even whinnied contentedly as we approached. But something new had been added. Above his feed bin, there was a brightly colored box with a hand-painted nameplate that read *Scat's Kathouse*. The cat didn't have to hide in the rafters anymore. He not only had a special place now, with comfy cedar-filled bedding—but just above the box was his very own heat lamp.

We stood there with our mouths open, as Phil said, "Well, what do y'all think about what we did here?"

"We're impressed. Scat's come home now. So Justice is calm and healthy." And I couldn't help but ask, "But for how long? What if this ol' tom decides to go roamin' and cattin' around again?"

Scat's tail curled and wagged a little, since he'd heard us. But he didn't move. He was purring at full volume while his front paws were kneading Justice's withers. With a wide yawn, his purring became even louder as he stretched out to the full length of his body. Laying there draped over the horse's back, with his front legs on one side and back legs on the other, he looked like a jockey's yellow saddle. Mavis burst out laughing, and began petting him. And Rich pushed the cat's tail to one side as though he were examining him. Scat drowsily raised his head, but his eyes remained half-closed.

Then picking the cat up and holding him in his arms, Rich announced, "Scat won't be cattin' anymore. He's been neutered...by Dr. Horton, I presume."

Natty grinned and even blushed a little, and Phil put his hand on his shoulder, saying, "Looks like it'll take awhile for Scat to get used to his own house. And it's possible he'll continue to prefer Justice's back. But at least we know he won't go out gallivantin' anymore.

"By the way, Mavis, Scat, Justice and I are going to Fort Worth together. How 'bout you doctors comin' along with us? Like Scat, my roamin' days are over, too. So I'd say it's high time for all of us to enjoy good friends...and heat lamps."

As we trudged back out into the soupy fog toward our vehicles, Mavis had the last word, as usual. Slapping Rich on the backside, she giggled, "You can learn something from this, boys. Cattin' around has its price. If y'all ain't home come bedtime...then your woman may seriously consider neutering as an option."

17

Piglet's Makeover

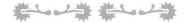

"Hurry, come over here and see this," gasped Rachel as she looked out the front window of Meadow Creek. Then when Tracy exclaimed "Ohmigod," Rich and I were too curious not to find out what was going on. It was odd to see both girls with their noses practically pressing against the windowpane.

Even Dr. Vest exhaled, "Whew...will ya look at that!"

A white stretch limousine had just pulled up in front of the clinic. It remained there for five minutes, its tinted windows hiding any possible peek at the occupants.

Limos of every color and size were a common sight in Dallas. But we were in the suburbs, and one had never pulled up in front of the clinic before. Even our wealthiest clients drive either Jeeps or pickups.

When frequent high-pitched sounds began emanating from within the elegant town car, Rich said, "Geeze...listen to that squeal. What is it?"

Suddenly, the rear door opened and who should step out from the leather interior but Doug Sanborn. Rachel caught her breath and couldn't speak. But our Tracy went into professional mode, saying, "Let's not all gawk like this. To your stations everyone. He's obviously goin' to come in here with a critter of some sort."

He stood waiting at the curb, looking as if he was still on the set of one of his movies. Even the silver hatband on the actor's wide-brimmed Stetson glinted in the sunlight. Realizing I was dating myself, I ended up saying, "He looks like Clark Gable...except he has bigger eyebrows. I read last week that he and his wife were comin' to live in Dallas. But what's he doin' out this way?"

The good-looking fellow held a thin leash and began walking toward our door. But whatever he had at the end of that tether wasn't about to leave the back seat. In his resonant baritone that was familiar to each of us, he coaxed, "Come on, boy." Finally, a cute pot-bellied pig slipped from the upholstery and onto the sidewalk. He was probably around four or five months old. But his baby squeals revealed that he wasn't too happy about this trip. Mr. Sanborn impatiently tugged on the harness-style leash, "Come on, Henry, you've got to see the nice doctor."

Henry obediently began walking a few steps until he came up to the dog-scented grass in front of the clinic. His tail curled tight, and his ears twitched. After a few sniffs with his snout, Henry froze. His short legs locked, and he sat down like a belligerent child. After pleading and cajoling a little more, the movie star threw up his hands in frustration, then bent down to pick up the resistant boar. Since we were still standing at the window, fascinated by this encounter, we scrambled to our normal positions to greet the celebrity and his frightened patient.

The actor had both arms wrapped around Henry, so Rachel ran over to the door and held it open for him, "It's a real pleasure to meet you, Mr. Sanborn," she sang out in her sweetest tone.

Rich and I had worked with our share of celebrities throughout the years, so we weren't so awestruck. "Howdy, Doug, I'm Dr. Vest and this is Dr. Carlton...whatcha got there?" asked Rich.

"My wife gave me this 'lil guy for my birthday...but I believe he has some problems. His skin stinks."

"Follow me to our exam room," I said, "...and let's see what we can do." I remembered the first time in vet school that I'd ever heard of this particular dermal condition. At that time, due to its name, I thought it had something to do with parakeets. I motioned for Rich to follow us. "Dr. Vest, it looks like Henry has 'parakeratosis'. Come on in with me because you won't see it very often. The symptoms are obvious and consistent...they never vary."

While Henry now sat quietly on the stainless table, he let me poke at him while I explained the condition to both

Doug and Rich. The round areas of abnormal patches on the pig's skin created crusty formations, and were part of the reason for the smell. "See those thick raised welts. It shows a zinc deficiency in Henry's diet...and too much calcium."

"I'm afraid we often feed him what we eat. And, since we're always on the run, that means a lot of junk food," explained Doug. "But that skin disease sounds bad."

"Not really, he's young enough to respond well to treatment." I reached into our cabinet for a special salve, "Just put this ointment on those inflamed areas once a day. And change his diet. I'll give you a list of good foods for pigs. In the meantime, here's a container of vitamins to add to his food. Mash two and stir in with his food every day for two weeks."

"That's it?" asked our newest resident. "What about his odor? Is there something we can do to improve his scent? He has a small part in my current picture...so I'll be taking him in with me every day. He's fun and has a lot of personality. But I'd like him to smell good for the rest of the crew."

After I told him the treatment would alleviate some of the problem, Rich also chimed in, "Neuter him, Doug...that'll help, too."

I agreed, "If he's going to be a pet, as well as a performer, that's what you'll want to consider relatively soon."

Still serious, Doug let us in on a little more family business. "If I castrate him, I'm not sure what I'd tell my wife. She says she's looking forward to having him sire piglets."

Doug's wife was Cassandra Weeks, the new anchorwoman for one of Dallas' television stations. Her new job opportunity was one of the reasons for their move here.

"Henry's a smart tyke and he'll be even better company when he no longer smells," added Doug. "We also have other animals at home...six dogs and five cats. Cassandra can't resist visiting the animal shelters without wanting to adopt every creature she sees. But we do have some great friends who come in and care for them while we're away at work."

"The process only takes a few minutes," said Rich.

"Well...you don't know my wife." Henry squealed and darted across the table to his owner's arms. The baby cried out again and again until Doug held him close under his tailored wool jacket. Patting him gently, the actor said, "Maybe another time, Doc...I just haven't got the heart right now." This fellow impressed me. Doug may have appeared larger than life on the screen, but, in reality, he couldn't have been nicer or more down-to-earth.

I'd always felt it was best to let owners off the hook from making immediate decisions. So I suggested, "Why don't we get Henry's skin condition under control first. We'll re-check him again in two weeks. Then, if you want, we can discuss the possible neutering. You'll have had a chance to talk it over with your wife by then."

While stroking Henry's ears, Rich picked him up to carry him out to the waiting limousine. Doug and I followed and chatted about the genealogy of this breed. I told him that though Henry was adorable and cuddly now, he could grow to an enormous size.

"We've just bought a big place with acreage in North Dallas. And we're thinking of getting some horses, as well. Even if he does get large, he'll still be part of the family."

I admired the fact that this couple had such love and concern for animals. And I realized that if they stayed in Dallas, we'd have many more critters as regular patients. So I needed to ask him, "Doug, you're quite a distance from us... how is it you came to our clinic?"

Smiling, he said, "We were referred to you by someone who wants to remain anonymous. Let's just leave it at that."

As Rich and I watched the limo roll away, we pondered on who, among our many friends and clients, could possibly know these high-profile media folks from Los Angeles. One of them must be hobnobbing among the greats of the movie or television industry. But we couldn't come up with a name. We were grateful, though, to whomever it was...because he or she was certainly adding some fine folks to our client list.

* * * * *

I knew Doug would be the type of responsible person to do exactly as we advised. When he brought Henry back two weeks later, the pig was looking great. All the spots were gone...and the makeup people on his set didn't have to use anything to cover them up anymore. For such a baby, using makeup in the first place may well have caused the dermal problem. But I didn't mention that fact.

"Cassandra agrees that we'll need to have Henry neutered, so can I leave him with you today for the procedure?"

"Actually, if you want him anesthetized, you could leave him with us. But, normally, no anesthesia is required... though Henry will have a few moments of discomfort. If you prefer, I can have this done in ten minutes so you can take him home today. You can either stay in here or in our reception area." Doug decided to wait outside and catch up on some script reading.

Tracy and I took Henry into our largest operating room, which was soundproof. During the brief surgical process, the piglet squirmed and kicked. And I was glad Doug didn't hear his two little squeals. When we completed the procedure, Tracy opened the door and I set Henry down. As soon as his tiny hooves touched the ground, he took off at the speed of light...racing down the hall, around the corner and into the reception area. Then, literally jumping into his owner's waiting arms, Henry pushed his head underneath Doug's jacket for comfort. Turning to me, Tracy said, "You know, I'm glad Doug knows how special pigs are. And he's right...they really are intelligent critters. Like the animal experts always say, they're sure a whole lot smarter than dogs, cats, or horses."

Our film-star client was thrilled that he could bring Henry back to his sweet-smelling household. Tracy even presented him with some special lotion from a well-known cosmetic company. She rubbed a little on the pig's soft skin.

It was lightly fragrant and natural, and had no chemicals that would irritate him. Even Henry seemed to like it as he lifted his head and kept sniffing in the air. He made a little chortling sound, which we translated to mean he was satisfied.

"Aside from my wife, there's one other person who's really going to appreciate this new fresh scent...my eight-year-old son. Scott prefers a futon in his room. It rests on the floor, so it's easy for Henry to climb up on the end of the bed... where he sleeps through the night. He's already gained a few pounds since we last saw you. But he's so playful and has such a sweet disposition that Scott enjoys having him there."

"That may work for the time being," I said, "But, mark my word, Doug, within the next two years, you're going to need two king-sized futons just to accommodate Henry alone."

* * * * *

A few months later, Tracy came waltzing in and excitedly announced, "Guess whose movie I saw last night?" Not waiting for an answer, she had to tell us, "Doug Sanborn's new western...and it's a terrific film with lots of suspense. Doug plays the town's sheriff, and he was his usual charming self. But our Henry was the real scene-stealer. He had to do all sorts of things like running and hiding. They even had him climbin' a ladder. I couldn't believe how cute he was. That 'lil piggy's a real pro!"

I wasn't sure I'd get to see the movie. But I could tell we were headed toward a future of some delightful—and unusual—moments with these show-biz folks and their pets. And I had to admit that I was looking forward to it.

18

Feline Revenge

Like the proud tabby that he was, Safari lounged comfortably on the exam table as though he came in to the clinic every day. He mewed softly and began rubbing his broad whiskered chin against the back of my hand. Scratching him lightly under his neck, I said, "Howdy, kiddo...what's up with you?"

While briefly scanning the medical chart, I turned to his young owner, whom I'd known since she was a toddler. "So, Judith, after nine years, Safari is *now* missing his litter box?" Judith Brooks adored this chubby cat. Her parents had presented him to her on her 16th birthday, just after the family's summer trip to Africa. And Safari had been at her side ever since.

Judith's folks were our long-time neighbors. So we watched the girl grow up into the lovely twenty-five-year-old woman who was now standing here, with a look of bewilderment in her hazel eyes. I thought to myself that she was much too cute to be in such a dither.

As Safari swished his fan-like tail from side to side, Judith complained, "Doc, I don't know what to think... Safari suddenly came 'unbroken'." I hadn't heard it expressed in quite that way before, but I understood what she meant. Safari gazed up at her, in serene innocence, and the dark mask on his face made him look like a wide-eyed raccoon. "He's not just missing the litter box...he's peeing wherever he wants to. Maybe I should consult a pet psychiatrist, like the one who has a television talk show."

Up until now, Safari had been a model cat-citizen, tidy, housebroken and always meticulous. For his first five years, he lived with Judith in her parents' home. And he continued his neat habits when Judith moved into her own apartment after graduating from the State University of Texas. So I quickly asked the young brunet a bunch of questions: "Have you noticed blood in his urine? Or has he been straining to go... or does he need to urinate frequently? Has his water drinking habits changed?"

"None of that, Doc...he's eating, drinking and acting perfectly fine as usual...except for this nasty behavior change."

I reached under Safari's belly to feel the distention of his bladder, and to palpate his pelvis region. I wanted to determine the size, shape, and thickness of the bladder wall. The cat remained indifferent to all my prodding and poking. His bladder was half-full, and he showed no signs of tenderness or discomfort. When tiny spots of urine appeared on the stainless table, I pushed his tail away to prevent the smearing of what seemed to be a normal sample, and asked Judith to hold him a minute. I wanted to fetch a dipstick to measure his ketone, protein and glucose levels. With one blot of the urinalysis reagent strip on the droplets, it was evident that there were no abnormalities.

For some reason, Judith blurted, "Maybe he's got a Valium deficiency." Since there was no such thing, the remark surprised me. I never thought anyone of her age would equate the synthetic drug Valium with a natural body chemical. As soon as I frowned, she realized it had been a strange thing to say.

"Why in the world would you say something like that? Have you been trying to sedate him? You should know better than to try something like that. It could be dangerous for any animal." I realized, then, that I was beginning to sound like her father. Since her dad and I were friends, it was always natural for me to feel paternal toward her.

Judith grew quiet...so I changed my tone. Forcing a slight chuckle, I said, "Before you resort to tranquilizing this sweet cat, let's see if we can find out the real problem."

Something here was not quite right. For no apparent physical reason, Safari was urinating when and where he chose. And it was a good guess that the cat's condition was psychogenic. Judith wasn't telling me everything.

"Is the litter box kept clean? Or have you changed to a different brand of litter? That can sometimes make a difference. Have you switched the type of carpet cleaners or sprays that you use? And did you move Safari's box to another location?" In response, the young woman said there had been no changes, so I continued. "Have you changed your job at the software company? Or has your work schedule been altered? What about noisy neighbors? Have you started wearing a new perfume?" I was looking for a pattern of disruption—apparently in vain.

Last, but not least, a final question hit the target. "Where, *exactly*, has Safari urinated?"

Blushing, Judith said, "Oh, that's the worst part. He goes on my bedspread...and, in my boyfriend's laundry basket. Those two places, mainly. If I didn't know better, I'd think he was doing it out of spite."

I assumed her reluctance to tell me this earlier was because she didn't want anyone—especially her mom and dad—to know that her boyfriend was living in her apartment. "You don't have to tell me anything if you don't want to. But it might help me to understand Safari's mood change if I knew how long you and your boyfriend have been together."

"Joe's been at my place for about two months. But we've been fighting a lot. And Joe and Safari don't get along too well. Joe's always scolding him just because the cat sleeps on the sofa...then Joe gets cat hairs on his clothes...but..."

I had to interrupt, "And, *how* long has Safari been acting out?"

"About two months," answered Judith, turning red again with sudden awareness. But then, she started giggling.

I joked with her by stroking my chin and pretending to be some wise old wizard. And I leaned over to talk confidentially into Safari's ear. "Well, Safari...do you think Judith needs a new boyfriend?"

The big, easygoing cat pushed his head against the young girl's arm, and Judith picked him up to cuddle him close. She whispered, "I've loved you a lot longer than I've even known Joe."

In my fatherly fashion, I told Judith that animals—like humans—have a strong, though not always obvious, reaction to any environmental change. And that it was up to her to make whatever adjustments, if any, might be necessary.

A couple of weeks later, I ran into her after she'd been visiting her parents, "How's Safari...is his problem still persisting?"

"Oh, Doc...I was going to call you. Safari's bedwetting is like Joe...no more. Our relationship wasn't working." Then, grinning, she added, "My cat may have been jealous, but he was also wise. Joe was never right for me...and Safari knew it long before I did."

Vets everywhere encounter this type of scenario all the time. Since my colleagues and I have been witness to so many of these cases, we often swap tales about the varied and eccentric ways pets can behave. Animals can't talk, so they act out their feelings of rejection, hurt, or displeasure at having a favorite routine changed. When Judith mentioned the pet psychiatrist, she was probably on the right track. Critters have an emotional depth and sensitivity that, regrettably, many owners tend to overlook.

My partner says he feels like a therapist most of the time. And, just a week ago, he met Gina, a seal-point Siamese who began wetting in the bathtub every day. After the usual probing, Rich found out that her owner had turned the litter box north and south, rather than east and west—though it remained in the same spot, against the same wall, and in the same utility room.

Then, last month, Rich had an appointment with Poker, the fussy Persian, who started urinating in Ryan Scott's gym shoes. It only happened after Ryan came home from college during his summer vacation. Apparently, Poker was trying to hide the new and unfamiliar smell, which the shoes had picked up from the closet of Ryan's dorm room.

And Dr. Horton told us that just before he left Utah, one of his clients brought in Corky, a miniature poodle. After a divorce, his owner returned to work as a fulltime teacher. But every evening, she'd come home to find an eight-inch, round hole in the carpet, and the living room drapes pulled down. In this case, neither the divorce nor the fulltime work was the problem. It ended up that Corky was reacting to a scented deodorizing powder that the teacher began using on the carpet and drapes. So the tiny dog was doing his best to destroy both.

The list goes on...and the sagas are usually funny and familiar. Hardly a day goes by that someone doesn't enter the clinic with a brand new lament about another method their critters have used to communicate their feelings. In one way or another—good or bad—they'll always tell you.

19

Hippocratic Oath

A call from the DPS wasn't good. I'd just arrived home in the early evening, and Karen was waiting anxiously. "The Department of Public Safety has been trying to reach you...there's been a trailer wreck somewhere on the highway. Horses were involved and we're all needed."

Noticing how exhausted I was, she added, "Sit a second, and I'll call Officer McClure right back, 'cause he'll know exactly where we should meet up."

My wife was a fifth-generation Texan and no stranger to horses. She managed the Los Alamosa Arabian Farm, and during the course of business rode at least twenty Arabians a day. I called her a 'barn rat' since she was constantly caring for horses and outfitting stables.

After reaching Stan on her cell phone, Karen spoke to him for only a few moments. "He's at the scene...and he says the accident is on I-35, just south of Lewisville. Apparently, this storm and the slick highways may have been the cause for a horse trailer to jackknife and flip over. I'll call Dr. Vest and Dr. Horton and tell them to get out there, too."

K.C. jumped into the truck with me, while Karen followed with a horse trailer. Ten minutes later, Stan McClure met us at the site of the over-turned van. Heavy rains clouded our vision. But emergency lights from the fire trucks and squad cars helped to light up the night.

"How many horses are here...and what's their condition?" I asked.

Pointing to the trailer with its nose down in the embankment, Stan said, "Four...that we know of. Two horses were thrown clear and, surprisingly, they're not hurt that much." Karen and K.C. quickly headed toward them. "But, Doc, there are two horses trapped in the trailer."

I ran up to one of the several firemen surrounding the scene, since they'd have details. "I'm Doc Carlton...what's the story here?"

The fire chief, Gary Sims, took me aside. "The truck's upside down in the ditch, and the tongue of the trailer is buried in the mud. Both horses are jammed in the nose of the trailer. One of them is dead...broken neck. His body has kept the mare's front legs pinned against the trailer wall. She's quiet, for the moment, so we can't tell how badly she's injured."

After pulling up alongside one of the police cars, Rich and Natty jumped out and raced over to join me. We followed the chief and his men through the wet grass.

Inspecting the wreckage with their power-beam flashlights, we could see that the situation was bad on many levels. The mare was prone to sudden eruptions of panic. She was also term pregnant, which would complicate the type of calming agent we hoped to use. But her jugular vein couldn't be reached through the side panels of the trailer. To top it all, gasoline fumes were filling the air signaling impending disaster. Since we were about to drop over with dizziness from the noxious vapors, one of the firemen handed us each a facemask.

Gary was quick to give us instructions, "Doctors, if one of you can heavily sedate her, then we can use the Jaws of Life to cut the trailer open...but we need to move fast." He pointed to me since, in this instance, it was good to be the small, slender one of the three doctors present. I didn't know why until a few moments later.

Along with three firefighters, I climbed on top of the rain-drenched trailer. And, with great care, we worked to pry open the bent and crumpled hatch door. It budged to an opening that was only a few inches around...just enough to insert a thin arm while lying on one's side. Through the vent window, I was able to view the mare's upper neck and the whites of her eyes. And though I was reaching blindly through the hole, I could feel her mane and stroke her. My heart went out to the mare. Her facial veins were dilated with fear, but her sudden onset of jerking and thrashing subsided when I touched her and spoke, "Whoa, girl...it's okay...whoa." When the mare nickered, I felt she sensed we were there to help her. I asked Rich to hand me a prepared syringe. While again soothing, "Whoa, now...," I used an 18-gauge hypodermic needle to inject the only protruding vein I could feel, knowing the strength of the solution would work within a few minutes.

No one wanted to holler, in case it spooked the horse even more. So, in a voice just above a whisper, Rich urgently exclaimed, "Hurry, Doc...you gotta get off of there. The fumes from the ruptured fuel tank are getting stronger." Checking on the mare's face through that side vent again, I saw that the strong medicine had taken effect. And I yanked my arm out from the hole a little too quickly, cutting it on the jagged edges of metal.

"Jump! Jump now!" Gary shouted, as I slid and tumbled to the muddy ground. Rich ran up, grabbed my arm to get me on my feet, and yelled. "Let's run...Run!" Everything happened fast as flames suddenly erupted. Immediately, the firemen were hosing heavy sprays of thick, white extinguishing foam showering us and the trailer. All I could see as we scrambled from the chaos was Karen standing at the top of the knoll. I knew what she must have been thinking. And, at least, I felt relieved that the mare had been knocked out before the blaze.

As a team, these firemen worked at jet speed. It was amazing to watch. They covered the trailer like ants...as water pumped, saws buzzed, and swift orders were relayed from one to the other. In the distance, I heard my son holler, "Dad...are you okay?"

Still dazed, I yelled back, "Yeah...I think so."

Then Karen cried out, "Look...look...oh, thank God!" I turned to see the rescue team dragging the pregnant mare to safety. The flames hadn't yet reached the inside of the trailer. But I could hardly wait to get over to her. I really needed to check on her condition and that of her unborn colt.

Natty emerged from the darkness to bring me up to date on the other two horses. "We calmed their nerves and treated the abrasions. And your wife already has them loaded into our clinic trailer."

"Hey, Doc...over here," Gary called out. The mare's leg is cut pretty bad."

Rich and I got to the mare's side, and Karen ran to fetch the necessary dressings. The mare's left forearm had suffered a deep gash, but we sewed several stitches to close the wound before she started to waken. "Rich, you can take the other two to the clinic...and I'll bring the mare in with Karen's trailer."

Sighing with exhaustion, Gary quietly said, "What a wreck this was, Doc...but we heard that Deirdre Mattix will be indebted to your whole group."

"Who?" asked Rich and I together.

"She's the owner. We just called the hospital to check on her driver. He has multiple injuries, including broken ribs...but he'll be okay. Anyway, after the ambulance had whisked him off, he had no way of knowing what happened to the horses. Overcome with worry, he asked the nurse to let us speak with him, so he could report back to the owner. He said he was enroute to Florida to bring these thoroughbreds to Ms. Mattix. And though it was a real tragedy to lose one, he was grateful that you were able to save that mare. She's an eight-year-old Arabian worth $250,000."

"We woulda done the same for one worth fifty cents," I commented.

"Amen to that," agreed Rich. "We'll be contacting Ms. Mattix to let her know when the three will be strong enough to travel again. And her stables can make new arrangements to pick them up."

Then he added, "But it isn't us that should be thanked. It's y'all...you guys with the hoses and the pickaxes and the nerves of steel. I know, 'cause my brother Danny's one of you. If it wasn't for you, we'd have seen a different ending here tonight."

20

Second Opinions

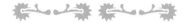

Squeezing every last second from the yellow light, I scooted Ol' Blue across the last intersection just a block before the clinic. I'd been weaving in and out of rush-hour traffic, but Tracy and I were still running late. I wouldn't be on time for the appointment with Clara Green and her pup. And Dr. Vest wouldn't be able to cover for me, since he was out on calls, too.

After sliding Ol' Blue to an abrupt stop, I asked Tracy to jump out and go tell Mrs. Green that I'd be right in. I needed to reach Karen to let her know I wouldn't be home again tonight...until late. She'd gotten the same message from me the day before, and the day before that.

For the past three days, we'd all been scrambling around the clock—blindsided by a highly contagious disease in the canine population. As people first started picking up sickly dogs from the side of the road, no one had an idea that it was just the beginning of what was to come. We were now in the midst of a 'parvovirus' epidemic. Newspapers ran stark headlines that read 'The Dog Killer'. Estimates were that, in the city alone, 15,000 or more animals each week would be afflicted during the coming months.

Our clinic could hold only eighty at one time...on a revolving basis. For days on end, we heard the same thing over and over, "He hasn't eaten in two days, and now he's got bloody diarrhea." We'd save one pooch, then lose two. We'd save three, then lose two more. We had no time to handle any interruptions. And our usual interactions with clients had to be limited, so their pets could be treated immediately.

As soon as I greeted Clara Green, I could see the lady was perturbed. Wearing a T-shirt with a 'Pets R Us' logo, the slender redhead looked worn and tired. Dark circles under her eyes indicated she'd been awake all night. This was another common sign among dog owners these days.

"It's about time you got here," she snapped. "I've been waiting for two damn hours."

Her tone startled me, and I tried to apologize. "I'm sorry we were twenty minutes late, but..."

Interrupting, she rudely gave an order. "I don't want to hear about it. Just take a look at my dog. His breath is bad, and his nose is hot."

Spike was in an obvious state of depression. The fur on his tan hindquarters was moist and soiled. And the rancid, characteristic odor was unmistakable. The German shepherd pup drooled bile-discolored saliva. As he rested his chin flat against the table's surface, Spike's eyes had an unfocussed, glassy look. His body and legs remained splayed out, since he had no energy to move.

Mrs. Green pushed the listless twelve-week-old across the table. His eyes moved a little and he stared at the blank wall. He whimpered weakly just as a gut-wrenching vomiting spell of stomach acids took hold of him. "He's been throwing up like that for two solid days," his owner said. I quickly moved to cover the sour fluids with paper towels, as Mrs. Green went on, "I'm a breeder. And I know when a dog is sick. He's got a fever, so I forced him to eat a warm mash of cottage cheese and honey. I know what to do."

The little guy had parvo. Infected animals were dying in the streets. If left untreated, the affect of the virus and toxins in the bloodstream would prove fatal. Everyone on our staff had calluses on their palms from swinging mops to disinfect the wards a dozen times each day. And blisters were forming on the tips of my fingers from threading I.V. catheters into the veins of all the others treated before Spike. But Mrs. Green's overbearing attitude hampered the necessary speed of care for her pup. Still, I continued to verify all the clinical signs, including serious dehydration from vomiting and diarrhea, low white blood cell count, and weakened heart muscles. And, again, the diagnosis was confirmed. But I wondered—as I did with every dog—if it was too late to stop the fast progression of the illness.

We were informed that researchers likened the disease to the cat distemper virus. And, though not verified, some thought the virus had mutated from the cat population. Many vets tried to use the feline vaccine as a preventive measure. But, for all the good it did, they might just as well have poured each dose on the ground. Clinics across the country were communicating with each other constantly. Scientists were doing what they could to combat the deadly organism that was known, but had never shown up in dogs until around 1978 when it began to appear in some northeastern states. Then it suddenly exploded here in Texas...and rapidly spread across the country. We were told, however, that an effective vaccination was imminent. In the meantime, constant hydration for infected dogs was imperative.

So we got ready. Picnic tables that would double as exam tables were purchased by each city in great numbers. They were set up in strategic parking lots that would become mass, emergency treatment centers. When the vaccine doses arrived, clinics across the state would be able to speedily administer the newly created antidote to thousands of pets at one time, as well as prevent healthy dogs from being exposed. Even physicians and medical practitioners volunteered to help out on a shift basis. It would be the largest full-scale plan for animals we might ever be witness to.

Until then, rows of I.V. bottles dripped life-supporting fluids to our kennel patients. And Spike needed to join them. I wondered how I'd convince Clara Green. She'd brought in a report of her own clinical treatment, which included two cat vaccine shots she'd given to Spike herself.

Tracy and Rachel stepped out of the room, knowing I was about to butt heads with Clara. Giving her the truth was the only way. This was no time for a debate. "Clara Florence Green," I said, "Spike has parvovirus."

The woman went through the roof, "*Tarbo?* That's not only impossible, but absurd. My dogs can't get *tarbo.*" Her face flushed red. "As I've told you, I'm a breeder...and I know all about *tarbovirus.*" I simply nodded as she raised her voice even louder.

"You're just trying to rip me off by giving Spike medicines that he doesn't need." I patiently folded my arms and continued to listen to her ranting, thinking that maybe it would make her feel better. And perhaps her hysterics were a way of covering up her fear. Young puppies from two to six months old were the most vulnerable to the virus. If she'd been giving Spike the ill-advised cat distemper shots, then she must have known a little of what was happening.

"Just give him a shot for the vomiting. I'll take care of him myself, because you don't seem to know anything!" With that, she grabbed Spike, saying "Gimme my dog!" And in a baffling emotional state, she stalked out of the clinic mumbling to herself.

* * * * *

Early the next morning, after going through the kennel wards, Tracy was perplexed. "Doc, what's Spike doing here in the hospital? I saw 'Mrs. Dog Breeder Who Thinks She's a Vet' storm out of here yesterday, never to return. She was going to treat the parvo herself, even though she can't pronounce the disease."

"I'm kinda rushing and can't talk right now...but maybe Rich can fill you in."

I overheard Rich say he'd keep the story short. "Last night, about 10:30 P.M., I was checking on the I.V. catheter that was flowing fluids sporadically to Mud Flap, our little cocker spaniel. I'd just finished when Clara called. 'You've got to meet me at the clinic immediately,' she said. 'I can't stop Spike's vomiting...he's throwing up volumes of brown, watery gunk'."

"Well," asked Tracy, "...what did you say to her?"

"I told her I'd meet her, but since it was after ten o'clock, I'd have to charge her the regular after-hours emergency fee."

"Oh, no...," exclaimed Tracy, "She must have blown her top!"

"You won't believe this, but she said, 'The hell you will. You sons of bitches are all alike...you're only in it for the money.'

"I bit my tongue, and said, 'Look lady...Spike has suffered from your ignorance long enough. If you want us to try and save your puppy, then meet Doc Carlton here at the clinic in thirty minutes'.

"Then, Tracy...I called Doc and told him that Mrs. Green finally agreed with his diagnosis, and she only wanted *him* to treat Spike."

"What a sneaky thing to do to Doc. You're impossible!"

Grinning, Rich added, "Yeah, I know...and poor Doc had to actually *pry* Spike from Clara's arms...at 11 o'clock. But the truth is that she should have left him with Doc in the first place."

* * * * *

Mrs. Green was defiant when I met her, since I was the last person in the world she wanted to see. But I was smiling and courteous, because I didn't know Rich had pulled another fast one on me. But, in her heart of hearts, she must have realized that at this point, she needed to trust someone, "Do what you must for Spike...but I still don't think it's *tarbo*." While I tended to the pup, she disappeared to use the phone at the front desk. On her return, she was abrupt again, "Well, that confirms it. I just talked to my friend, another breeder, and she said the consensus among other breeders is that Spike couldn't possibly have *tarbo*."

As I taped Spike's catheter in place and adjusted the flow of his supportive drip, I mumbled, "That's good...I'm relieved to hear it."

"And, he doesn't have bloody diarrhea."

I administered another injection and whispered to myself, "Just wait a day..."

"I heard that...and I don't have to wait. I know!"

I wondered where this woman came from. And, why now, in the midst of this emergency when everyone was bending over backwards to cooperate. Hadn't she seen the papers with articles appearing daily alerting folks to the complexities of this virus? We knew so many knowledgeable

breeders who were doing a great service. But then there were
a few, with no medical training, who set themselves up as
experts, only to end up putting animals at risk.

It was almost midnight, and Clara was still lecturing
me...until I gave her a firm 'look'. She quieted while I carried
Spike into the isolation ward. On the front of his cage, I hung
a liter of fluids marked 'Parvo Golden Juice' and said, "These
electrolytes will replace what he's lost." And on the cage card,
I wrote PARVO in red letters—a mandatory procedure when
contagion is present.

Gasping, Clara demanded, "Erase that now. How many
times do I have to tell you that he doesn't have *tarbo*."

"No, ma'am, he doesn't have *tarbo*. In fact, I don't even
know what that is."

Mrs. Green went stomping out of the kennels, yelling
at me over her shoulder, "I'll have you know that I'm a highly
respected canine breeder. And if my dog dies because of your
misdiagnosis, I'll sue your ass off!"

I still couldn't believe Rich had set me up again. But
I laughed to myself, realizing I'd done the same to him a few
weeks before, when I sent him out alone to the Tumbleweed
Farm to dehorn 'a few calves'. It turned out to be more than a
hundred calves.

Throughout the night, Spike's condition continued to
decline. Though, in the early morning, his vomiting subsided.
But behind his rear legs floated a pool of bloody diarrhea. The
puppy could barely lift his head. I washed the stench from

his fur. And his drained body felt limp as I carried him to another clean cage.

Later that morning, Tracy handed me Spike's blood counts. In spite of my efforts, the results showed severe hypoglycemia and lymphopenia. Damn, I thought. The pup's blood sugars and cellular defenses were too low. And there was nothing else I could do except to hook another I.V. on line, and hope Spike would fight to survive.

"Keep the fluids flowing during the rest of the day, Tracy. That's Spike's only chance now. Maybe we can outrun the virus."

* * * * *

Strangely, two days passed and we hadn't heard anything from Clara Green. Against all odds, Spike slowly rallied and began to nibble on a few morsels of food, which he was able to keep down.

Though Clara hadn't contacted us, half the vets in town had called. The first was Dr. Phil Stemo from the Denton Clinic who asked me how the parvo dog was doing.

"Which one? There's forty of 'em back here."

"That's what've we've got here, too," he said. "I'm talking about Spike, the angry lady's dog. Clara Florence Green called me at 4:00 A.M. two nights ago, then again last night. I told her Spike didn't have *tarbo*, because there's no such thing...and that she was probably thinking of parvo."

"Would you like a referral, Phil?"

"No thanks!"

"Who called next?" asked Rich.

"Dr. Eric Tomis from the Hill Street Hospital. And he was more direct."

"Doc, how's that parvo dog, Spike? And who's this witch that called me six times. Find some way to stop her. I don't have the patience for her nonsense." Then he hung up.

Tracy intervened, "Yeah, that's when Dr. Jerry Waters from the Grapevine Clinic called. He was the third in two hours."

Rachel hollered out, "Here's another doctor on the Parvo Hotline, Dr. Jim Foyt."

"Doc Carlton, are you treating Mrs. Green's dog for parvo? She's called me four times in two days...including at 6 o'clock this mornin'."

"Shoot, Jim...that's doin' good because she called Dr. Stemo at 4:00 A.M. And she contacted Dr. Tomis six times... so guess we're makin' some progress. Spike's been here in the hospital for three days. So, would you like a referral, Jim?"

"Hell, no," he answered. "I've got enough problems."

This time Dr. Vest reached for the ringing phone, and it was Clara. As soon as I got on the line, she blurted out, "I now have second opinions on Spike's case. I've been consulting with several veterinarians, and they all agree with me..."

In the most pleasant voice I could conjure up, I said, "Then, Mrs. Green, you may wish to call Dr. Stemo, Dr. Tomis, Dr. Waters, and Dr. Foyt one more time. I regret to say this, but what they said and what you heard are two very different things."

Stuttering a little, Clara swiftly changed the subject, "How is Spike doin'?"

"It's been touch and go...and we want to watch him closely. But we're pleased that he's beginning to respond and starting to eat. The diarrhea has also stopped. He's still extremely weak. But it looks like your little guy will recover."

I thought she'd be thrilled by the news. But she suddenly reverted back to her old self. "It wasn't *tarbo*, ya know..."

"Yes, ma'am, I know."

"I'm a breeder, and I..."

"Yes, ma'am, I know...you told me. Your wonderful puppy can go home the day after tomorrow. I'm sure that will make you very happy. So we'll see you then...on Thursday." I was still wondering why the woman remained so confused by the name of the virus. I thought that maybe, like a lot of folks, she was just dyslexic. And perhaps she didn't realize it or didn't want to admit to it. Whatever the reason, at least Spike would recover and, hopefully, someone who wasn't as obsessive as Clara would adopt him.

Just then, Rachel announced, "Mrs. Victor just got off the line. Her cow is having problems delivering the calf. So I told her someone would be out to her place within fifteen minutes. Then Katy Noel called. She's coming in right now with her three dogs. They haven't been able to eat in two days, and one has bloody diarrhea."

Rich shuddered, "When will this epidemic end? How much longer?" He knew the answer as well as I did.

"They tell us that cases of vaccine vials will arrive shortly. So, hopefully, we can control this bug in another month or so. But it's apparent that parvovirus is here to stay. It'll be more common than distemper. But, in the future, we'll at least be able to vaccinate our dogs early...and keep the incidence of infection to a minimum.

"Right now, I need to get out to Mrs. Victor's farm. And I'll take Billy with me so Tracy can stay and help you. I should be back in time to relieve you tonight, but we'll call you from the road to see how Katy's three dogs are doin'. Sure hope they'll be as lucky as Mud Flap and Spike."

21

What's in a Name?

I t was already late in the day, and it looked like another rainstorm might be rolling through. Mrs. Victor's place was just outside of town, so I figured our visit wouldn't take long. For months, Billy had been begging to go on farm calls, and now was as good a time as any. He'd been putting in long hours during the crisis, and needed a break. In his second year of college on an athletic scholarship, he was still working in our kennels part-time. We often had him bouncing between both clinics, since he was willing to do anything. He also had his sights set on getting into veterinary school after graduation.

Slowly rolling through the city in bumper-to-bumper traffic, we had little to do but listen to the latest news on the dog epidemic and gaze at the surroundings. To my eye, there was nothing to see in Dallas but a multitude of glass skyscrapers. The sight always had a way of putting me in a reflective mood, "Billy...see those two corporate towers over yonder? I can remember when that whole area was an ol' cow pasture."

But Billy's thoughts were elsewhere. A red convertible, full of tanned, longhaired pretty girls, pulled up alongside us. Their rock 'n' roll was on high volume, and they were almost dancing out of their seats. Our college boy smiled at them, "Hey, Doc...look at the driver. She's gorgeous." The light changed and the bevy of beauties pulled away, still giggling and waving.

I went on talking, probably more to myself than to the sophomore athlete. "Guess I didn't realize how much Dallas had changed until the other night when we all went out to my once-favorite restaurant. I was the only fella there wearing a cowboy hat, boots, and jeans. Did you notice? I had on a sports coat...but the other gents had on three-piece business suits. There wasn't a hint of Texas in that whole room of diners. They were eating steaks, but I had the feeling that most of those folks had never seen a cow."

I'm sure Billy hadn't heard a word I said. Though he exhaled with a "Whew!" when we passed the entrance of one of Dallas' many gated communities. Sprawling three-story homes were sequestered behind tall, vine-covered stone walls. "Geeze, Doc, how can anyone afford these homes. What could these people possibly do for a living?"

"Well, they sure ain't veterinarians," I laughed, "...and they can't all be drug dealers. I'd guess they're corporate execs,

lawyers, bankers, and 'real' doctors. But I don't rightly know."
I had the feeling, then, that Billy may never become a vet.

The skies opened up and the rains pelted down on us.
Billy tried to read Rachel's directions. But, in her scribble, all
we could make out was that Justine Victor's place was a wood-
frame farmhouse with white trim. If we came to a Catholic
church on a hill, it would be on the west side of Renner Road.

Ol' Blue's windshield wipers beat out a rhythm to the
rain like a metronome. Low, greenish clouds swirled down
to touch the ground in front of us—and thunderous claps
reverberated through the air like sonic booms. My headlights
were useless. Streaks of lightning bolts flashed across the treetops,
and fast rising waters rushed to fill the low spots on the road. By
now, we should have been somewhere in the area of the farm.
Then, in the distance, a small light moved back and forth. Mrs.
Victor must have been waving her kerosene lantern to mark the
direction we should take up the muddy trail.

We got to the fence of her property line—actually
three broken boards hanging from a single hinge on a cedar
post. Standing there in a hooded poncho, Mrs. Victor
signaled us to stop. At her feet was a cluster of metal cans.
She was using them to identify the end of the hollow pipe
that funneled the rising run-off alongside the asphalt road.
Following her lead, I turned to cross over the drainage, sliding
Ol' Blue into the slick, sandy loam.

I'd seen the ageless woman twice before in Noble's
general store, but we never really met. I'd heard she was a
long-time widow—gritty, tough, and set in her ways. Billy

cracked open the window, shielding his face from the rain, and asked, "Are you Justine Victor?"

"Hell, son, who else would be out in this gawd-damn storm?" Pulling open the truck door, she grumbled while cussing a blue streak and wiped her eyes with the back of her hands. Climbing in, she pushed Billy over toward me, shaking water from her yellow poncho onto the floorboards. Slumping down low in the seat, she let out a "Whoo-eee, damn nice f···in' weather we're havin'. Ain't it? I can't believe June Bug chose to have her damn calf on this frog-stranglin' evenin'." Her boots were muddy, and her dark hair was plastered wet to her head, but the gold tooth in the center of her broad smile was 'pure Justine'. She was just as I remembered: short, pudgy and vocal. She cussed like a barroom parrot, and didn't mind if anyone cared. Every few sentences were punctuated with a word beginning with 'F'.

"Last year, June Bug calved in a snow storm...and now, this. Why that f···in' heifer's goin' to be the death of me yet," she said as she punched Billy's shoulder for emphasis. "Drive straight ahead, Doc, June Bug's in my f···in' barn...if it ain't washed away yet."

I couldn't make out anything in the blackness, but kept Ol' Blue plowing up one knoll and down another. I'd slow down and squint to see, waiting for flashes of lightning to give us visibility.

We slithered to a stop in front of the so-called barn, and Justine and I hopped out. Water poured down in sheets from the wood-slatted roof. And open cracks leaked heavily

into the room-size lean-to. Bales of hay were stored in each
end of the small dilapidated shed. As hailstones began to
pound against the rotten planks, I spotted June Bug in the
far corner, circling around and around at a frantic pace.
Her nostrils were flaring and her eyes were crossed by the
labor pains. In order to block the nervous cow's escape, Mrs.
Victor had created a makeshift metal gate that was hastily
wired between two posts. I hollered at Billy to maneuver and
manage the light beams from the truck so the barn could be
illuminated for our work. June Bug's hooves were tromping
knee-deep in the muck, and steam rose from her sweat-laden
back. At the sound of an earth-shaking thunderclap, June
Bug bellowed loudly and spun around. That's when I saw two
small feet hanging out from the cow's vulva. "No wonder June
Bug's wild and afraid. This ain't good!" I hollered out.

"Whelp...let's just get 'er done," Justine yelled back.

The heifer went ducking into the shadows for safety.
Apparently, the farmer lady's abrasive shouts and the look of
her wind-flapping poncho spooked the delirious bovine even
more than the thunder had.

"C'mon, Justine...let her settle down a bit," I urged.

Mrs. Victor cursed, "It's the f···in' hail that's got 'er
riled. Can you rope 'er?"

I called to Billy to toss out my lariat from behind his
seat. I caught it midair, just as my boot soles sank down into
the sticky soil. Easing through the openings of the wired
barrier, I gathered a loop. As I sloshed toward June Bug, the
boggy mixture of straw and slush gripped my every step with

the thickness of wet cement. June Bug now had her head buried in the corner. When I approached, she snorted but didn't spin around. On my third loop, I snagged her horns. A quick jerk on the rope held securely. But when I reached to wrap it around the center post of the shed, I lost my balance and went down hard. Wiping mud from my elbow, I sat in the wet muck.

As I went scrambling on my knees toward the pole to try again, the anxious cow glared at me on the ground and a vapor cloud of humidity escaped from her mouth as she began huffing. "Uh, uh...this is definitely not good!"

"Doc, watch out! She can be meaner than a one-eyed badger," warned Justine.

Too late...a sudden crackling blast from the heavens ignited June Bug into a charging frenzy. Her hooves snapped out of the mud, her horns went down and her thousand-pound body lunged toward what she probably thought was the reason for her pain—*me!*

I slid belly first, bobsled-style, trying to dodge her rage. But, again and again, she furrowed the soaked ground as she pawed with her massive forequarters...ready for another strike.

"Why you ol' bitch!" screamed Mrs. Victor. "He's here to help ya."

By this time, Billy had bounded out of the truck, and stood there calling out, "What can I do? What can I do?"

"Do *anything* to divert her attention...or wave something in front of her," I choked out.

Before June Bug could surge forward again, I managed to get some slack from my lariat's dally. I pulled backwards with a firm grip on the rope, gaining a few inches in our tug-of-war.

"You've almost got 'er," encouraged Justine. "Pull, Doc...pull." As her horns drew nearer to the pole, I placed my foot on the center post and struggled to snub June Bug's brow to a still position.

"Once more," urged both Billy and Justine in unison.

Searing my palms on the twisted lasso for the last time, I finally got the rope tied snug. "There," I grunted, "...now we can begin the work we came for."

Justine sang out, "We did it!" as she jumped up and down like a geriatric cheerleader.

With June Bug's horns now tied to the base of the pillar, I was able to stand. But the cow's hindquarters were planted in the mud, suddenly frozen in contractions. Her heavy breaths came quickly. Concerned about the calf, I lifted the heifer's tail.

"The little one's still alive!" exclaimed our excited client.

After examining the calf's condition, I wanted to swear myself, "Dang...those were the *back* feet. I'm going to have to turn the baby around. The calf is upside down and backwards."

Needing to gather strength and to figure out the best thing to do, I climbed back through the gate and stood outside in the refreshing rain for a few moments of quiet.

Covered with the filth from the shed's muddy floor, I smelled bad. I stepped under the barn's overhang where the waters poured down so I could shower with my clothes on, while chipping gunk from my hair and coveralls. Billy handed me the surgical soap, and I scrubbed my hands and arms as best as I could. It may not have been totally sterile, but we couldn't be picky at a time like this.

Determined, I took a deep breath, and went back inside, "Well, the calf's gotta come out."

Considering June Bug's advanced labor and all the energy she'd just used up, I didn't think she'd be able to remain standing for long. As I began to reach inside her, her back legs splayed. Then she slipped and fell on her side. She scrambled to stand, but fell. Then she'd try again, only to fall again. Finally spent, she quieted. As she lay on her side, I decided to try and position the calf. On my stomach, with both arms buried in the cow's reproductive track, I maneuvered the term fetus. Afterbirth fluids ran down the front of my coveralls and my skin was soaked with mucus and slime. I flopped around in the slush, like a fish on a muddy embankment, while sweat rolled into my eyes. Straining, I tried to rotate the body of the unborn baby.

The force of June Bug's uterine contractions complicated my efforts. The pressure of her muscles mashed my forearms against her pelvic bones, and my fingers went numb. Between the cramping, I was finally able to grasp the calf's nostrils, and grip the forelegs. With all the strength I could muster, I flipped the torso, head and forequarters into the pelvic canal. Wrapping the O.B. chains around the forelegs, above the knees and ankles of the baby, I tugged and pulled, "We're almost there, Justine. Ask Billy to hand me the calf-jack...he'll know what it is."

Billy quickly pushed the cumbersome tool toward me, as I assembled its parts and prepared to extract the wedged infant.

"I wanna help, too," said Mrs. Victor, "Just gimme a minute." Then she started to climb over her rickety gate.

The barn creaked and shifted, and I joked, "Don't knock the shed down, now."

"This ol' barn is studier than an iron horse," she exclaimed.

Every muscle in my body ached. But with our obstetrical device in place, each turn on the lever smoothly guided the emerging newborn out into the world. June Bug bellowed during this final release. And, like a rowing coach, Justine enthusiastically led each turn of the handle by chanting, "Stroke...stroke... stroke."

When I felt the calf's hips clearing the pelvis, I smiled and looked over to Justine.

"Well, I'll be horn-swaggled...he's alive!" yelled Mrs. Victor as the slippery calf and I went sliding against the wall in a pool of amniotic secretions. June Bug let out a groan of relief, while I tried to hold her baby's face out of the muck.

The woman was so overcome with glee that she spun around in a circle, "I worried that June Bug would be a bitch to save. But, you did it, you f···in' did it, Doc. She sure as hell had a gawd-damn fine baby bull."

"Yep...she sure did!" chuckled Billy.

Justine's joy was contagious. And I couldn't help but laugh with her. I set the newborn down on a dry patch of dirt, saying, "Stay right here, boy, while I see if your mother's okay."

June Bug was unusually quiet. She tried to get to her feet, but couldn't make it. She called to her calf, and the hungry calf cried back. After what she'd been through, it appeared that the new mother had some pelvic nerve damage. I'd seen it before, but was still worried. Extracting the baby applied such tremendous pressure inside the pelvic canal that her major nerves were temporarily bruised. With rest, she'd walk. But June Bug wanted to be with her calf. Suddenly the big cow partially stood, but her back legs buckled under her. She fell backwards, pulling the lasso tight and uprooting the shed's center post to which she was tied.

Justine screamed, "Look out...duck!" I grabbed for the calf, as the shed began to sway back and forth. The lean-to pitched and rocked violently as we tried to scramble out. But, with a thunderous upheaval, it collapsed on top of us.

After a moment of quiet...I heard Justine coughing in the dusty aftermath. "Is everyone okay?" she hollered.

Since he'd been near the door, Billy had gotten out. He dashed in to pick up the debris that surrounded Justine. "We're fine, too," I yelled, as I sat there between two rafters... still holding the startled baby across my lap.

"What about June Bug...how's my Juney?" Justine asked anxiously.

I tried to explain, "I don't know yet...but she might be okay 'cause it looks like those tall bales of hay took the brunt of the force, keeping the main part of the roof from hitting us."

Billy cleared the splintered timbers away from me, and I was able to look around for June Bug. Some fallen wood planks shifted and through the dusty haze, I saw June Bug's shoulders move. Still holding the calf in my arms, I made my way over to her. She didn't appear hurt, though she was covered with broken boards. The tip of her tail twitched, but there didn't seem to be any cuts on her hide. She lay there almost relaxed...showing no fear whatsoever. Her ears slapped away the falling drops of rain. She looked at me and blinked her eyelashes, but didn't move another muscle. Heaving deeply, the cow let out an enormous sigh. I grabbed a handful of hay and put it in front of her. She took it quite contentedly, and the sound of her teeth grinding on the parched steams told me that all was right with the world.

Billy was about to remove the rubble covering June Bug, so I could lay the calf next to her. But the hail began to come down again. And he stayed with June Bug, continuing to pull away the shed fragments. I snubbed the calf's pink muzzle against my chest and, stepping over broken slats, quickly carried the newborn to the cab of Ol' Blue to prevent him from being pounded by falling balls of ice.

"Justine, let's wait in the truck 'til the worst of the storm passes by. June Bug's safe, and Billy's working to remove the rest of the barn's remains from around her." Just then, Billy ran to the truck, grabbed a canvas sheet and then ran back. After he'd made some sort of temporary tent protection for the stunned cow, he joined us.

The three of us, and the wet young bull, waited there, scrunched together, for an hour. With the windows rolled up, it smelled like a gym locker inside. But no one seemed to mind. Mrs. Victor held the small bovine, removing bits of mud from his ears and hooves...and tears rolled down her face. Our vents were emitting warm air. So she nestled the squirmy infant in front of them, and announced, "I'll call him 'Carlton' after you, Doc."

Though totally drenched and exhausted, I was still happy for June Bug and 'Carlton'. In spite of the bizarre circumstances, we'd done everything medically possible. When the storm quieted, we each helped to free June Bug. And, as if nothing had happened, she retracted her back legs to her belly and stood with ease. She snorted to her calf and gently began licking the baby dry and nursing him. The youngest bovine, with milk still dribbling from his lips, uttered a satisfied *baaaaaa.*

We gathered up our equipment and loaded Ol' Blue, while Justine turned up the radio full blast, and warmed her bones at the heater. She was beaming with pride as she watched June Bug and Carlton begin to meander back to her small herd of three steers, four goats, and six chickens.

Shaking a spray of water from the soggy brim of my hat, I said, "Well, it's time for us to go home. But keep in touch, 'cause we'll want to know how y'all are doin'."

Mrs. Victor snapped off the music. And, in the sudden silence, the irrepressible woman said, "I surely do appreciate all your kick-ass help, Doc." Then the not-so-tough old character gave both Billy and me a rib-busting hug.

As we made our way back out over and through the muddy ruts, bumping and jostling all the way to the main road, we looked back to see Carlton prancing in the drizzle. With his heels kicking up, it was great to see him being playful...as though he'd had a normal birth.

It's not likely I'll ever have a street or a college named after me. But, somehow, having my name given to the offspring of a cantankerous ol' heifer seems an honor—and only fitting. Because no matter how much time goes by, or how many of those skyscrapers soar up around me, only one fact remains: I am now—and always will be—a die-hard country vet.